Infection Control and Safety: A Guide for Healthcare Providers

Mark Zelman, PhD
Associate Professor, Biology
Aurora University

Carrie L. Milne-Zelman, PhD
Associate Professor, Biology
Aurora University

PEARSON

Boston Columbus Indianapolis New York San Francisco Upper Saddle River
Amsterdam Cape Town Dubai London Madrid Milan Munich Paris Montréal Toronto
Delhi Mexico City São Paulo Sydney Hong Kong Seoul Singapore Taipei Tokyo

Publisher: Julie Levin Alexander
Publisher's Assistant: Regina Bruno
Editor-in-Chief: Marlene McHugh Pratt
Executive Editor: Joan Gill
Associate Editor: Melissa Kerian
Editorial Assistant: Stephanie Kiel
Development Editor: Rose Foltz
Director of Marketing: David Gesell
Marketing Manager: Katrin Beacom
Senior Marketing Coordinator: Alicia Wozniak
Production Project Manager: Debbie Ryan
Senior Media Editor: Matt Norris
Media Project Manager: Lorena Cerisano
Creative Director: Jayne Conte
Interior Designer: Dina Curro
Cover Designer: Suzanne Behnke
Cover Photo: Centers for Disease Control and Prevention
Project Management and Composition: Revathi Viswanathan/PreMediaGlobal
Printing and Binding: R.R. Donnelley/Crawfordsville
Cover Printer: Lehigh-Phoenix Color/Hagerstown

Library of Congress Cataloging-in-Publication Data
Zelman, Mark.
  Infection control and safety : a guide for healthcare providers / Mark Zelman, Carrie
   L. Milne-Zelman.—1st ed.
     p. ; cm.
  Includes index.
  ISBN-13: 978-0-13-304566-6
  ISBN-10: 0-13-304566-8
  I. Milne-Zelman, Carrie L. II. Title.
  [DNLM: 1. Health Personnel—Problems and Exercises. 2. Occupational Health—education—Problems and Exercises. 3. Infection Control—Problems and Exercises. 4. Safety Management—Problems and Exercises.
5. Universal Precautions—Problems and Exercises. WA 18.2]
  LC Classification not assigned
  363.15—dc23   2012036953

10 9 8 7 6 5 4 3 2 1

Notice: The author and the publisher of this volume have taken care that the information and technical recommendations contained herein are based on research and expert consultation, and are accurate and compatible with the standards generally accepted at the time of publication. Nevertheless, as new information becomes available, changes in clinical and technical practices become necessary. The reader is advised to carefully consult manufacturers' instructions and information material for all supplies and equipment before use, and to consult with a health care professional as necessary. This advice is especially important when using new supplies or equipment for clinical purposes. The authors and publisher disclaim all responsibility for any liability, loss, injury, or damage incurred as a consequence, directly or indirectly, of the use and application of any of the contents of this volume. Many of the designations by manufacturers and sellers to distinguish their products are claimed as trademarks. Where those designations appear in this book, and the publisher was aware of a trademark claim, the designations have been printed in initial caps or all caps.

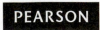

ISBN 13: 978-0-13-304566-6
ISBN 10: 0-13-304566-8

BRIEF CONTENTS

CONTENTS

PREFACE

We are pleased to present the first edition of *Infection Control and Safety: A Guide for Healthcare Providers*. We hope you will agree that this engaging and accessible text presents current, credible, and relevant information about best practices in infection control, chemical safety, and radiation safety in the healthcare workplace. The text supports courses in clinical and laboratory safety, supports continuing education workshops and seminars, and serves as a professional reference for healthcare professionals. Written in a personal style, the text is well-supported with references and resources as well as handy tables and charts that highlight key infection control as well as chemical and radiation safety concepts, facts, procedures, and regulations.

The text takes a comprehensive view of safety hazards facing healthcare workers. Topics include agencies and standards pertaining to infection control and safety, infectious diseases and healthcare-associated infections, blood-borne pathogens, prevention, and postexposure prophylaxis. In addition, chemical and radiation safety are addressed, providing an overview of best practices that are integral for safety in the healthcare workplace. Appendices expand related supporting topics, including nationally notifiable infectious conditions, healthcare-associated infections, and reproductive health hazards. Case studies in each chapter challenge the reader to apply the material to realistic scenarios in healthcare. Chapters are also supplemented with *Words of Warning!* and *Work Safe!* boxed features that highlight special infection control and safety topics. Each chapter includes authoritative resources and references.

REVIEWERS

Hanaa Guirguis, Hanaa Guirguis, M.B., CH. B., CCMA, CPT1
National Career Education
Rancho Cordova, California

Kris Hardy, CMA
Brevard Community College
Cocoa, Florida

Dolly Horton, CMA, M.Ed
Asheville Buncomber Technical Community College
Asheville, North Carolina

Lucinda Hunsberger, CMA
YTI Career Institute
Mechanicsburg, Pennsylvania

Michelle Mantooth, MSC, MLS (ASCP) CM, CG (ASCP) CM
Trident Technical College
North Charleston, South Carolina

Jose Sanchez, MD, AHI (AMT)
ECPI University
Virginia Beach, Virginia

Amy Semenchuk, Dean of Academics
Rockford Career College
Rockford, Illinois

Paula Silver, PharmD
ECPI University
Virginia Beach, Virginia

Lynn Slack, BS, CMA
Kaplan Career Institute, ICM Campus
Pittsburgh, Pennsylvania

ABOUT THE AUTHORS

Mark Zelman, PhD, is Associate Professor of Biology at Aurora University in Aurora, Illinois. A native of Chicago, Mark received his BS in Biology at Rockford College. Mark received his PhD in microbiology and immunology at Loyola University Chicago and was a postdoctoral fellow at University of Chicago, where he studied molecular cell physiology. Mark draws upon years of practical experience and formal training in infection control and safety. During his tenure as biology professor, research scientist, and college administrator, Mark developed and implemented laboratory safety and chemical hygiene plans for several institutions. Mark pursues a wide range of interests in biology, enjoys bird-watching and camping with his family, and wears out quite a few running shoes each year.

Carrie Milne-Zelman, PhD, is Associate Professor of Biology at Aurora University in Aurora, Illinois. Carrie earned her BS in Biology and Mathematics at Alma College in Alma, Michigan. She received her PhD in Genetics from Iowa State University and was a National Science Foundation postdoctoral research fellow in bioinformatics at Indiana University. Carrie has many years of experience teaching biology lectures and laboratories to prenursing, health science, and biology undergraduate students. She enjoys hiking, camping, and bird-watching with her family.

CHAPTER 1

Introduction: Principles and Practice of Safety

This chapter describes the rationale for learning and practicing infection control and safety in the healthcare workplace. Key concepts, terminology, practices, and resources related to infection control and safety are also introduced.

Objectives

After completing this chapter, the student will be able to:

- Describe the benefits of maintaining a safe healthcare workplace.
- Explain the chief types of hazards faced by healthcare workers.
- Name key laws designed to protect health and safety in the healthcare workplace as well as the agencies that oversee and enforce these laws.
- Understand how engineering controls, safe work practice, administrative controls, and personal protective equipment prevent healthcare workplace hazards.

Key Terms and Concepts

administrative controls
blood-borne pathogen
chemical hazard
engineering controls
healthcare-associated infection (HAI)
infectious disease

Occupational Safety and Health
   Administration (OSHA)
personal protective equipment
radiation hazard
safe work practice

The Importance of Workplace Safety

Rewards and challenges await you as you provide healthcare and its many supportive, critical services for patients. Population growth and changing demographics ensure that growth in healthcare fields will continue to outpace most careers in the United States. These careers require dedicated, well-educated professionals who are trained in the science and technology of their fields. Effective healthcare professionals recognize that infection control and safety also form the foundation of their practice because a safe workplace protects employees and patients, and improves the quality of patient care.

The modern healthcare workplace provides a variety of services ranging from highly specialized to comprehensive. Thus no one description can accurately portray your working environment. Healthcare roles comprise many types of positions (Table 1-1 ■). Healthcare professionals provide a variety of patient services such as diagnosis, treatment, health screening, preventive services, and recordkeeping. Some professionals work with infectious microorganisms, handle hazardous chemicals, or administer x-ray examinations, while others provide vaccinations or assist with medical and surgical procedures. Healthcare positions are diverse and include medical office assistants, surgical assistants, dental hygienists, medical laboratory technicians and scientists, radiologic technicians, physical and occupational therapists, and massage therapists.

Reducing Exposure to Hazards

Healthcare employees face potential health hazards in the workplace, regardless of their position or whether they provide patient care directly or indirectly (Table 1-2 ■). Patients, too, are at risk. Perhaps the most obvious of these health hazards is the risk of acquiring or transmitting **infectious diseases**. Diseases caused by microorganisms may be transmitted from person to person. For example, respiratory diseases such as influenza and tuberculosis are spread by respiratory droplets from one person to another. Other microorganisms are carried in blood and thus are called **blood-borne pathogens**. These include the viruses that cause hepatitis and AIDS. Specific infectious diseases are transmitted through characteristic routes. (See Chapters 3, 4, and 5 for detailed discussions of infectious diseases and blood-borne pathogens.)

TABLE 1-1. The Diversity of Healthcare

Healthcare Services	Healthcare Workplaces	Healthcare Professionals
Diagnosis	Outpatient clinic	Medical office assistant
Treatment	Outpatient surgery	Surgical assistant
Screening	Hospital	Dental hygienist
Prevention	Community clinic	Phlebotomist
Recordkeeping		Radiologic technician
		Medical laboratory technician
		Physical therapist
		Occupational therapist
		Massage therapist

TABLE 1-2. Hazards in the Healthcare Workplace

Type of Hazard	Examples
Infectious	Tuberculosis, influenza, staphylococcal skin infection, urinary tract infection, HIV/AIDS, hepatitis B, hepatitis C
Chemical	Skin, eye, and respiratory irritants; flammable, explosive, corrosive, and/or carcinogenic chemicals
Radiation	Immune suppression, mutagenic, carcinogenic effects, low birth weight, miscarriage, birth defects

The scope of **healthcare-associated infections (HAIs)** is staggering. The Centers for Disease Control and Prevention (CDC) reports that approximately 1.7 million infections are acquired annually in healthcare workplaces in the United States. These HAIs lead to 99,000 deaths each year. Fortunately, properly and universally employed infection control procedures significantly reduce the transmission of infectious disease in healthcare workplaces. For example, infection control procedures such as hand hygiene and use of gloves and masks greatly reduce the incidence of all types of catheter-associated infections, common HAIs.

Chemicals in the healthcare workplace also pose many types of health hazards (Table 1-2), and attention must be given to storing, dispensing, and disposing of them safely. Some **chemical hazards** are widespread, and many healthcare professionals may not recognize them. For example, glutaraldehyde is a widely used disinfectant and a skin, eye, and respiratory irritant. But products containing glutaraldehyde bear different trade names, underscoring the importance of employee training about labels and hazardous chemicals (Figures 1-1 and 6-3). Exposure to hazardous chemicals can be reduced by following **Occupational Safety and Health Administration (OSHA)** recommendations for storage, ventilation, use, personal protective equipment, and disposal. OSHA, under the U.S. Department of Labor, prescribes that most workplaces using hazardous chemicals develop and implement a chemical hygiene and safety plan to protect workers. (See Chapter 6 for a detailed discussion of chemical safety.)

Radiation exposure is also hazardous to health. Employee exposure to **radiation hazards** can be virtually eliminated by attending to safe work practices and using appropriate protective equipment. (See Chapter 7 for a detailed discussion of radiation safety.)

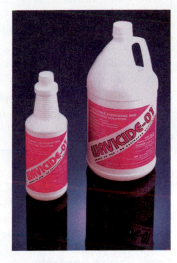

FIGURE 1-1.

Glutaraldehyde is a hazardous disinfectant with many different trade names. *Source*: Medical Chemical Corporation (MCC).

The Safe Work Environment

Safe working environments emerge from collaboration between employers, employees, and regulating agencies. Several agencies oversee workplace safety. Primary among them is OSHA, which prescribes safety standards regarding hazardous chemicals, blood-borne pathogens, personal protective equipment, radiation, and other areas. The roles of OSHA as well as other regulatory agencies and standards are described in Chapter 2.

Safety standards alone do not protect employees and patients from workplace health hazards. Employers must put these standards into practice, enforce them, and train employees. In turn, employees have the right to know the hazards as well as how to protect themselves and their patients. Furthermore, employees are responsible for learning and adhering to applicable standards.

WORK SAFE!
A Safe Workplace Is Your Right and Responsibility

The Occupational Safety and Health Act (OSH Act) requires employers and employees to reduce or eliminate hazards in the workplace. The OSH Act states that each employer (1) shall furnish to each employee a place of employment free from recognized hazards that are causing or are likely to cause death or serious physical harm and (2) shall comply with occupational safety and health standards promulgated under the act.

Each employee shall comply with occupational safety and health standards and all rules, regulations, and orders issued pursuant to the act that are applicable to his or her own actions and conduct.

Several elements of a safe working environment plan interact to protect employees and patients. These elements include **engineering controls**, **safe work practice**, **administrative controls**, and use of **personal protective equipment** (Table 1-3 ■) and will be discussed throughout the text.

Engineering Controls

Engineering controls focus on eliminating biologic, infectious, chemical, and physical hazards from the work environment. Safety experts consider engineering controls to be the most important factor in workplace safety because these controls do not rely on

TABLE 1-3. Infection Control and Safety Plan Elements

Plan Element	Examples
Engineering controls	Ventilation, air filtration, chemical hood, UV lighting, negative pressure work room
Safe work practice	Employ best practices, follow documented procedures and standard operating procedures, use PPE when required, use standard precautions, use aseptic technique
Administrative controls	Written plan, written standard operating procedures, defined responsibilities, incident reporting procedure, recordkeeping, inspection, training
Personal protective equipment (PPE)	Use gloves, respirators, masks, gowns, protective eyewear, leaded aprons, and other PPE when required

Source: Occupational Safety and Health Administration www.osha.org

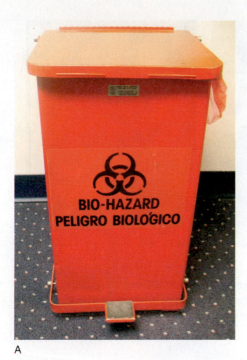

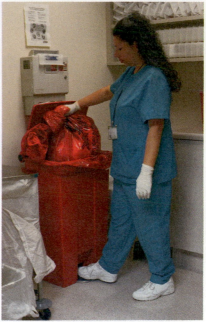

A   B

FIGURE 1-2.

Biohazard storage is an engineering control. (A) The container is clearly labeled, impermeable, and accessed by a foot pedal. It isolates biohazard waste from employees and patients. It should be conveniently located near the site of waste generation to minimize waste transport. (B) A healthcare worker safely disposes of a biohazard bag. *Source*: (A) CDC/Kimberly Smith, Christine Ford and (B) Smith, *Clinical Nursing Skills*, 8e, p. 440, lower right.

human choice or judgment and generally cannot be thwarted by human error. Several specific engineering controls will be discussed in this text. The principles behind these controls include the following:

Design: Create facilities, equipment, and work processes that eliminate hazards. For example, the facility floor plan should not require employees to walk through labs to access employee dining areas, and biohazard storage should be placed adjacent to areas where biohazards are used or generated, eliminating unnecessary transport of wastes (Figure 1-2).

Substitution: Replace a hazardous substance or procedure with one that is not hazardous. In x-ray facilities, digital x-rays can replace the need for glutaraldehyde, a hazardous chemical used to develop x-ray film. Mercury thermometers should be replaced by digital or alcohol-based thermometers.

Segregation: Separate people from hazards, create barriers between people and hazards, and enclose hazards. For example, contaminated needles, biohazards, and chemical waste should be stored in a safe place in secure containers (Figure 1-3). Ventilation and chemical hoods are also examples of engineering controls (Figure 1-4).

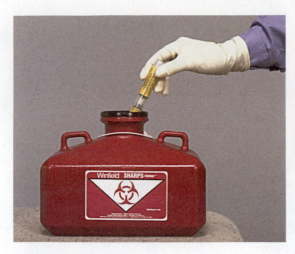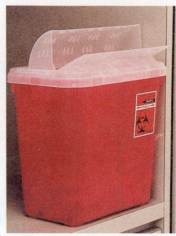

FIGURE 1-3.

Sharps containers. These impermeable containers must be marked with the biohazard symbol and be available at all locations where needles are used. They must be operated with one hand and be located at convenient height, never on the floor. *Source*: Michael Heron/Pearson Education.

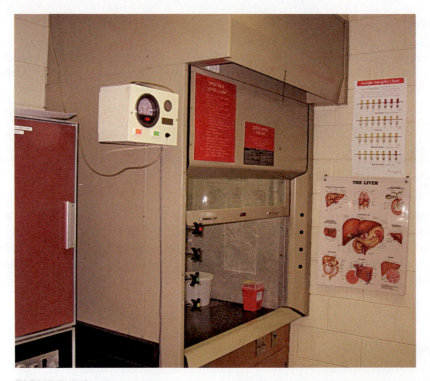

FIGURE 1-4.

Biologic safety cabinet. These cabinets contain splashes and small droplets generated when working with pathogens. *Source*: Karen Kiser, William Payne, Terry Taff.

Maintenance: Repair or replace faulty equipment and machinery. Clearly, ultraviolet (UV) lamps (which control pathogens on surfaces), ventilation, or sharps containers are of no use if they are not in working order.

Safe Work Practices

Employers establish safe work practices. These rules and procedures direct employees on how to safely perform their duties. By following these practices, employees provide a higher level of safety and further reduce exposure to hazards. Many safe work practices are required by specific OSHA standards.

Administrative Controls

The employer establishes administrative controls, a set of work procedures and safe work practices. The employer should distribute and enforce written safety policies, designate supervision of safety programs, maintain records, and train employees. Examples of administrative controls include the following:

- Perform maintenance on hazardous equipment when staff will not need the equipment, preferably when staff is not working at all, to reduce exposure to hazards.
- Monitor worker exposure to ionizing radiation.
- Reduce clutter and minimize chances for accidents.
- Establish procedures for storage and disposal of hazardous substances.
- Label chemicals and post signs that identify known hazards (Figure 1-5).
- Provide employee training on safe work practices.

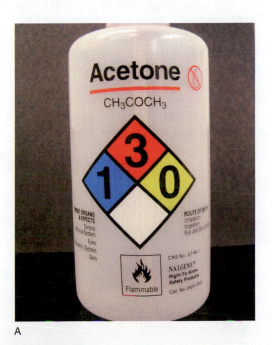
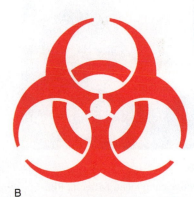

A   B

FIGURE 1-5.
Chemical hazard label and biohazard sign. Administrative controls include signs and labels.
(A) Chemicals must be properly labeled to communicate hazards. (B) Signs must be posted
to identify known hazards. *Source*: (A) Karen Kiser, William Payne, Terry Taff (B) CDC.

WORDS OF WARNING!

Read for Safety

Your employer will probably post signs, labels, safety information, and safe work instructions throughout the workplace. None will be effective if you do not take the time to read them, ensure you understand them, and work accordingly. In particular, you must:

- Read and follow warnings on all chemical labels.
- Read and adhere to all posted warning signs.
- Read and follow all safe work practices provided by your employer.
- Follow all directions for safe work practices.
- Get training on the correct use and fit of all personal protective equipment.
- Know and follow all infection control measures in your workplace.

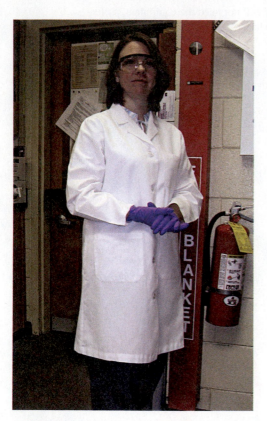

FIGURE 1-6.

Personal protective equipment. Different PPE is required under different circumstances. PPE includes gloves, protective eyewear, and gowns. *Source*: Karen Kiser, William Payne, Terry Taff.

Personal Protective Equipment

Engineering controls, safe work practices, and administrative controls may not eliminate certain hazards. In such a case, personal protective equipment (PPE) is required. PPE does not eliminate hazards, so employers and employees must understand that if PPE is not used or if it fails, people will be exposed to the hazards. Employers must assess the workplace for PPE needs. OSHA's PPE Hazard Assessment and Training standard specifies how to assess the workplace and implement PPE training. Employers must match each type of PPE to the specific hazard, maintain PPE, make PPE readily available, and provide regular training on PPE use. PPE includes gloves, masks, gowns, leaded aprons, goggles, and respirators (Figure 1-6).

Chapter Summary

- The modern healthcare workplace offers diverse services that are provided by a variety of healthcare professionals.
- Employees and patients face potential hazards in the healthcare workplace.
- A safe working environment is a right and responsibility.
- A safe working environment improves patient care.
- Agencies and resources support safe working environments.
- Preventing workplace hazards involves engineering controls, safe work practices, administrative controls, and use of personal protective equipment.

Application

Case Study 1-1: Why Infection Control and Safety Matter

As the senior medical office assistant with many years of experience, you are frequently asked to orient new employees. While touring the clinic with a newly hired medical office assistant, you brief the new employee on infection control procedures such as hand hygiene and vaccination. The new employee seems surprised and asks why the office is so worried about infections.

Questions:

1. Explain why it is important that you and the other medical office assistants take precautions to prevent infections.
2. When answering the new employee's question, what resources can you provide to support your reply and provide additional information?
3. What can you do if the employee remains unconvinced about the importance of infection control?

Case Study 1-2: Identify Elements of a Safe Working Environment

Services at your clinic include venous blood draws (phlebotomy) for various diagnostic and preventive healthcare purposes. As you show the new medical office assistant around the facility, you point out a sharps container for used needles, a biohazard container, and a hand hygiene station with alcohol hand rub. You explain how and when gloves, gown, and mask should be worn. You explain the importance of attending training workshops on blood-borne pathogens. You also show the new employee how and when to complete the injury and incident report form. Afterward, you tell the new employee about the following incident, which resulted in a colleague's exposure to blood-borne pathogens: While cleaning a room, the custodian picked up paper towels that had been left on the counter. Wrapped up in the paper towels was a used syringe that punctured the custodian's hand. The sharps container was nearby on the counter and it appeared to be full.

Questions:

1. Which type of control measure failed in this situation: engineering, safe work practice, administrative, or PPE?

2. What steps should be taken to avoid this kind of accident in the future?

Assessment

Select the one best answer.

1. Which of the following is considered the most important type of safety control?
   a. administrative
   b. work practice
   c. engineering
   d. personal protective equipment

2. Gloves, gown, mask, and respirator are examples of _____.
   a. administrative controls
   b. work practice controls
   c. engineering controls
   d. personal protective equipment

3. Fume hoods, biosafety cabinets, and sharps containers are examples of _____.
   a. administrative controls
   b. work practice controls
   c. engineering controls
   d. personal protective equipment

4. Which is a component of administrative controls?
   a. ventilation
   b. safety training
   c. gloves
   d. vaccinations

5. Which is a component of safe work practice?
   a. standard operating procedures
   b. ventilation
   c. safety training
   d. gloves
   e. vaccinations

Resources

American Chemical Society www.acs.org
American Conference of Governmental Industrial Hygienists www.acgih.org
American National Standards Institute www.ansi.org
Association for Professionals in Infection Control and Epidemiology www.apic.org
Bureau of Labor Statistics Occupational Outlook Handbook www.bls.gov
Centers for Disease Control and Prevention www.cdc.gov

Clinical and Laboratory Standards Institute www.clsi.org
Department of Energy www.doe.gov
Food and Drug Administration www.fda.gov
Joint Commission www.jointcommission.org
National Institute for Occupational Safety and Health www.niosh.gov
Nuclear Regulatory Commission www.nrc.gov
Occupational Safety and Health Administration www.osha.gov

PEARSON
myhealthprofessionskit™

Visit www.myhealthprofessionskit.com to access the interactive Companion Website for this textbook. Simply select "Basic Health Science" from the choice of disciplines. Find this book and log in using your user name and password to access additional learning tools.

CHAPTER 2

Safety Resources: Laws and Agencies

This chapter describes key occupational safety laws, emphasizing standards set by the Occupational Safety and Health Administration (OSHA), and discusses other agencies and organizations that provide guidelines for safe practices in the healthcare workplace.

Objectives

After completing this chapter, the student will be able to:

- Describe the role of OSHA in maintaining safe working environments.
- Describe key OSHA regulations pertaining to the healthcare workplace.
- Name the major organizations and agencies that provide guidelines for chemical, biologic, and radiation safety.
- Describe the chief elements of a safety plan for the healthcare workplace.

Key Terms and Concepts

American National Standards
    Institute (ANSI)
blood-borne pathogens
chemical hygiene plan
Clinical Laboratory Improvement
    Amendments (CLIA)
CLIA-waived Tests
Department of Energy
U.S. Department of Labor
exposure control plan
hazardous chemicals
hazard communication

ionizing radiation
Nuclear Regulatory Commission
occupational hazard
OSHA Occupational Safety and Health
    Administration
Occupational Radiation Protection
standard operating procedures
Standards for Protection against
    Radiation
standards

Occupational Hazards

Work environments can present various **occupational hazards**. At worst, working conditions may cause fatalities. More common, however, are occupational injuries, infections, and diseases that result in lost workdays and short-term or permanent disability. The most recently available data show that hospital workers have a far higher number of occupational illnesses than many other occupations, including other selected healthcare positions (Table 2-1 ▪).

Keep in mind that each illness may involve an hour, a day, weeks, or months of missed work. The U.S. Bureau of Labor Statistics reports that occupation-related illnesses and injuries cause a median of 5 to 7 missed workdays among healthcare workers. These numbers represent a considerable loss of industry productivity, decreased quality of workers' lives, increased worker disability, increased employer expenses, and a great deal of healthcare costs. Protecting workers from hazardous working conditions is imperative.

Laws Protecting Healthcare Workers

Fortunately, employers have no choice in matters regarding safety: laws require them to take certain steps to guard against workplace hazards. By prescribing minimum standards and holding employers responsible, laws ensure that employee safety does not depend on employer judgment, whim, or level of interest. An examination of relevant laws, governmental agencies, and nongovernmental organizations (NGOs) is necessary to understand the foundation for safe workplace practices.

The Occupational Safety and Health Act

The Occupational Safety and Health Act (OSH Act) of 1970 guarantees the right to safe working conditions. The OSH Act gives workers rights and assigns employers responsibilities to ensure that working conditions do not pose a risk of serious harm to workers. Table 2-2 ▪ and Figure 2-1 outline these rights and responsibilities.

TABLE 2-1. Incidence Rate of Nonfatal Occupational Illness, 2008

Industry	2008 Average Employment, Thousands	Incidence Rate per 10,000 U.S. Workers				
		Total Cases	Skin Diseases or Disorders	Respiratory Conditions	Poisonings	All Other Occupational Illnesses
General medical and surgical hospitals	4,273.3	58.8	9.0	7.7	0.2	41.4
Ambulatory healthcare services; includes physician offices	5,643.1	22.9	3.6	3.1	0.2	16.0
Medical and diagnostic laboratories	220.3	12.7	1.1	3.7	—	7.9

Source: Occupational Safety and Health Administration Statistics www.osha.gov

TABLE 2-2. Workers' Rights under the OSH Act

Workers have the right to:

- Receive information and training about hazards, methods to prevent harm, and the OSHA standards that apply to their workplace. The training must be in a language they can understand.
- Observe testing that is done to find hazards in the workplace and get test results.
- Review records of work-related injuries and illnesses.
- Get copies of their medical records.
- Request OSHA to inspect their workplace.
- Use their rights under the law free from retaliation and discrimination.

Source: Occupational Safety and Health Administration www.osha.gov

The **Occupational Safety and Health Administration (OSHA)**, a division of the U.S. **Department of Labor**, was created by Congress under the OSH Act to set and enforce **standards** for worker safety. These standards are federal laws listed in title 29, section 1910 of the Code of Federal Regulations. Actual workplace practices may be more, but not less, stringent than federal law; thus these laws are appropriately called standards. Certain OSHA standards apply to certain workplaces because different workplaces present different hazards. Table 2-3 ■ describes the OSHA standards that apply to most healthcare workplaces. Later chapters explain how these standards are implemented in the workplace (Figure 2-2).

Blood-borne Pathogens Standard

Among the most important standards for healthcare workers, the Bloodborne Pathogens Standard aims to prevent occupational exposure to blood or other potentially infectious materials, such as body fluids or used needles that may contain blood. This standard is designed to prevent transmission of pathogenic microorganisms that are present in human blood, especially hepatitis B virus (HBV) and human immunodeficiency virus (HIV). These microorganisms are known as **blood-borne pathogens**.

Central to this standard is the requirement for a written **exposure control plan**. An exposure control plan is described in greater detail in Chapter 5, but here are such a plan's key elements:

- Identifies employees with potential for exposure
- Describes engineering controls and work practices, including the provision of hand hygiene facilities, sharps storage, and **standard operating procedures (SOPs)** for collecting, handling, storing, and disposing of specimens
- Describes how the employer will make available personal protective equipment (PPE) and hazard containment equipment
- Describes training available for proper use of PPE and hazard containment equipment
- Describes exposure follow-up procedures and recordkeeping
- Describes hazard communication, signs, labels, and related training (Figure 2-3)

In practice, detailed SOPs and guidelines for infection control are spelled out by organizations and agencies such as the Centers for Disease Control and Prevention (CDC) and the Association of Professionals for Infection Control and Epidemiology. Best practices in infection control are discussed in Chapter 4, and best practices in blood-borne pathogen safety are described in Chapter 5.

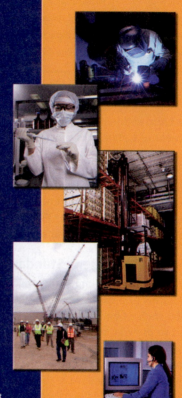

Job Safety and Health
It's the law!

OSHA
Occupational Safety
and Health Administration
U.S. Department of Labor

EMPLOYEES:

- You have the right to notify your employer or OSHA about workplace hazards. You may ask OSHA to keep your name confidential.

- You have the right to request an OSHA inspection if you believe that there are unsafe and unhealthful conditions in your workplace. You or your representative may participate in that inspection.

- You can file a complaint with OSHA within 30 days of retaliation or discrimination by your employer for making safety and health complaints or for exercising your rights under the *OSH Act*.

- You have the right to see OSHA citations issued to your employer. Your employer must post the citations at or near the place of the alleged violations.

- Your employer must correct workplace hazards by the date indicated on the citation and must certify that these hazards have been reduced or eliminated.

- You have the right to copies of your medical records and records of your exposures to toxic and harmful substances or conditions.

- Your employer must post this notice in your workplace.

- You must comply with all occupational safety and health standards issued under the *OSH Act* that apply to your own actions and conduct on the job.

EMPLOYERS:

- You must furnish your employees a place of employment free from recognized hazards.
-
  You must comply with the occupational safety and health standards issued under the *OSH Act*.

This free poster available from OSHA –
The Best Resource for Safety and Health

Free assistance in identifying and correcting hazards or complying with standards is available to employers, without citation or penalty, through OSHA-supported consultation programs in each state.

1-800-321-OSHA
www.osha.gov

OSHA 3165-12-06R

FIGURE 2-1.

OSHA requires that this poster be displayed in the workplace to inform workers and employers of their rights and responsibilities under the law. *Source*: http://www.osha. gov/pls/publications/publication.AthruZ?pType=Industry

TABLE 2-3. OSHA Standards That May Apply in Healthcare Facilities

Standard Title	Description
Occupational Exposure to Hazardous Chemicals in the Laboratory	Applies to all employees engaged in the laboratory use of hazardous chemicals as defined in the standard.
13 Carcinogens	Applies to the 13 carcinogens listed in this standard; applies to manufacturing, processing, repackaging, release, handling, and storage.
Blood-borne Pathogens	Applies to all occupational exposure to blood, potentially infectious materials, and all pathogenic microorganisms that are present in human blood; these pathogens include hepatitis B virus (HBV) and human immunodeficiency virus (HIV).
Ethylene Oxide	Applies to all occupational exposures to ethylene oxide (sterilizing gas).
Formaldehyde	Applies to all occupational exposures to formaldehyde, that is, from formaldehyde gas, its solutions, and materials that release formaldehyde.
Standards for Protection against Radiation	Applies to workplace exposure, monitoring, communication and warning, protective procedures, records, and reporting.
Ionizing Radiation	Applies to workplace exposure, monitoring, communication and warning, protective procedures, records, and reporting.
Hazard Communication	Ensures evaluation of hazards of all chemicals; transmission of information concerning their hazards to employers and employees; comprehensive hazard communication, including container labeling and other forms of warning, material safety data sheets, and employee training.

Source: Occupational Safety and Health Administration statistics www.osha.gov

---

WORK SAFE!
Your Workplace Safety Plans

In any healthcare workplace, whether outpatient surgery or a community vaccination clinic, you need to know, understand, and always use safe work practices and standard operating procedures. Your employer must provide these in an appropriate workplace safety plan, such as a blood-borne pathogen exposure control plan, a radiation exposure control plan, or a chemical hygiene plan. If you have any questions, you must ask your employer—and keep asking until you get answers.

Needlestick Safety and Prevention Act

The Needlestick Safety and Prevention Act of 2000 modified the Bloodborne Pathogens Standard to address exposure to needles and other sharps in the healthcare setting. The act requires employers to identify, evaluate, and implement use of safer medical devices, especially the various types of needles frequently used in the healthcare workplace. Employees must be involved in evaluating and choosing new needles and other devices. The act also requires employers to maintain a sharps injury log.

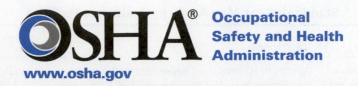

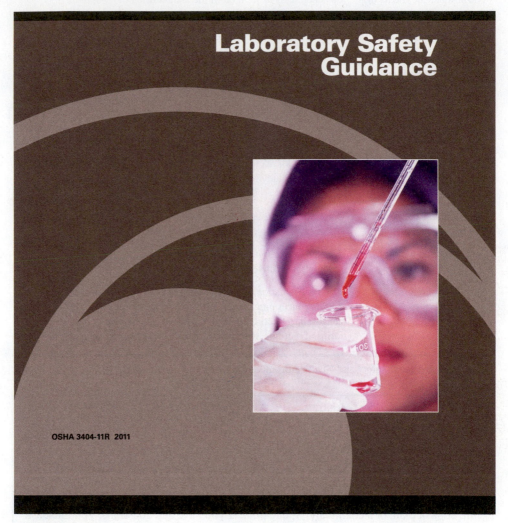

FIGURE 2-2.

In addition to prescribing standards, OSHA provides many educational publications and fact sheets on nearly any occupational safety and health topic. *Source*: www.osha.gov

Clinical Laboratory Improvement Amendments (CLIA)

The **Clinical Laboratory Improvement Amendments (CLIA)** guide clinical laboratory testing for diagnosis, screening, and treatment of human disease. The aim of CLIA is to provide standards to regulate the quality of laboratory testing. To ensure appropriate patient care, this testing must be performed accurately and safely. Thus many laboratory tests must meet CLIA standards. However, the CDC and the U.S. Food and Drug Administration (FDA) have determined that certain tests are so simple and routine that little risk for error exists. These tests qualify to be **CLIA-waived Tests.** They include tests such as glucose monitoring, urine dipstick tests, and color-based pregnancy tests.

Clinical Laboratory Standards Institute (CLSI)

Formerly called the National Committee for Clinical Laboratory Standards, the Clinical Laboratory Standards Institute (CLSI) develops standards for best practices and safety for clinical laboratories.

Occupational Exposure to Hazardous Chemicals in the Laboratory Standard

The Occupational Exposure to Hazardous Chemicals in the Laboratory standard applies to all employers that use **hazardous chemicals** in a laboratory setting. These hazardous chemicals are listed in the standard, which requires employers to implement a written **chemical hygiene plan** to protect employees from occupational exposure. The chemical hygiene plan must be available to all employees and must contain certain elements (see Chapter 6 and www.OSHA.gov for details).

Standards exist for certain hazardous chemicals that may not apply to all healthcare workplaces. For example, OSHA standards for carcinogens, ethylene oxide, and formaldehyde apply only to workplaces where these substances are present (see Table 2-3). Each standard defines the permissible limits for exposure, provides for the monitoring of employee exposure, requires the designation of regulated areas where exposure is expected, requires employers to provide respirators and to train employees in their use, and describes a plan for communicating hazards, labels, signs, training, and recordkeeping.

Hazard Communication Standard

The **Hazard Communication** standard focuses on all aspects of hazard communication. It requires employers to evaluate the workplace for the presence of hazardous chemicals; transmit information concerning these hazards to employees; and implement comprehensive hazard communication, including container labeling and other forms of warning, material safety data sheets (MSDS), and employee training (Figure 2-4). Thus this standard is a good resource for developing chemical hygiene plans.

The OSHA standards described here serve as the foundation for best practices in chemical safety. These safety practices are detailed by other organizations and agencies and are described in Chapter 6.

Radiation Standards

Healthcare workers may have occupational exposure to **ionizing radiation** from x-rays, cancer treatment, and other sources. **Standards for Protection against Radiation** (from the **Nuclear Regulatory Commission**) and the OSHA Ionizing Radiation standard define limits of workplace

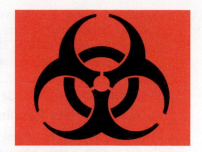

FIGURE 2-3.
OSHA standards require hazard communication and training. Employees should be trained to use and recognize this sign that warns of the presence of biological hazards. *Source*: Centers for Disease Control Public Image Library CDC/Henry Mathews.

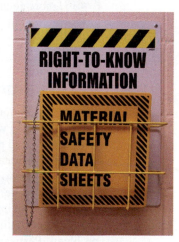

FIGURE 2-4.
Safety and health information, such as material safety data sheets (MSDS) about chemicals, must be readily accessible to workers at all times. *Source*: Travis Klein/ Shutterstock.

exposure, prescribe monitoring procedures, require means of hazard communication and warning, require protective procedures, and provide for recordkeeping and reporting. In addition, a workplace may follow the **U.S. Department of Energy** standard, **Occupational Radiation Protection**. Radiation standards and safety practices are described further in Chapter 7.

WORDS OF WARNING!
Common Safety Pitfalls

How many of us become absorbed in our work and forget to attend to our surroundings? Do certain tasks become so routine that you hardly think about them? Do you plan your work as carefully as you can every time? Gaps in safety often arise when attention fails. Avoid common pitfalls by following these guidelines.

Always
- Read the label of a container before using the contents.
- Read and follow standard operating procedures.
- Know and use the proper PPE.
- Ask questions if any confusion arises.
- Report spills, exposures, and accidents to supervisors.
- Report mechanical failure of any equipment.
- Report failure, shortage, or absence of safety equipment and PPE.
- Properly dispose of needles and chemical, biologic, and radiation waste.

Never
- Recap needles.
- Ignore signs and labels.
- Ignore equipment failure.
- Ignore failure, shortage, or absence of safety equipment and PPE.
- Eat, drink, or smoke in areas where these activities are forbidden.

Enforcement, Fines, and Filing Complaints

OSHA jurisdiction includes private sector employers and excludes self-employed workers, family farm workers, and government workers, except in those states that use other OSHA-approved plans. OSHA approves and monitors 27 states that use such plans; these plans cover private and public sector employees.

Workers who feel their workplace safety or their OSHA right to a safe working environment are being compromised may contact OSHA confidentially with questions or to file a complaint (see Figure 2-1). The regional OSHA officer discreetly investigates complaints, which sometimes involves site investigations, and directs employers to correct problems. Persistent safety violations can result in employer fines.

OSHA workplace inspections can occur unannounced. They also occur in response to employee complaints about sites that pose imminent danger. Violations can result in penalties, depending on the category of violation. Penalties may be $7,000 for each serious violation and up to $70,000 for each willful or repeated violation.

Confidential complaints can be filed three different ways:

- Online: A complaint form is available at http://www.osha.gov/pls/osha7/eComplaintForm.html.
- Fax: The complaint form can be faxed to the local OSHA regional or area office, which can be found at http://www.osha.gov (Figure 2-5).

U. S. Department of Labor
Occupational Safety and Health Administration

Notice of Alleged Safety or Health Hazards

For the General Public:

This form is provided for the assistance of any complainant and is not intended to constitute the exclusive means by which a complaint may be registered with the U.S. Department of Labor.

Sec 8(f)(1) of the Williams-Steiger Occupational Safety and Health Act, 29 U.S.C. 651, provides as follows: Any employees or representative of employees who believe that a violation of a safety or health standard exists that threatens physical harm, or that an imminent danger exists, may request an inspection by giving notice to the Secretary or his authorized representative of such violation or danger. Any such notice shall be reduced to writing, shall set forth with reasonable particularity the grounds for the notice, and shall be signed by the employee or representative of employees, and a copy shall be provided the employer or his agent no later than at the time of inspection, except that, upon request of the person giving such notice, his name and the names of individual employees referred to therein shall not appear in such copy or on any record published, released, or made available pursuant to subsection (g) of this section. If upon receipt of such notification the Secretary determines there are reasonable grounds to believe that such violation or danger exists, he shall make a special inspection in accordance with the provisions of this section as soon as practicable to determine if such violation or danger exists. If the Secretary determines there are no reasonable grounds to believe that a violation or danger exists, he shall notify the employees or representative of the employees in writing of such determination.

NOTE: Section 11(c) of the Act provides explicit protection for employees exercising their rights, including making safety and health complaints.

For Federal Employees:

This report format is provided to assist Federal employees or authorized representatives in registering a report of unsafe or unhealthful working conditions with the U.S.Department of Labor.

The Secretary of Labor may conduct unannounced inspection of agency workplaces when deemed necessary if an agency does not have occupational safety and health committees established in accordance with Subpart F, 29 CFR 1960; or in response to the reports of unsafe or unhealthful working conditions upon request of such agency committees under Sec. 1-3, Executive Order 12196; or in the case of a report of imminent danger when such a committee has not responded to the report as required in Sec. 1-201(h).

INSTRUCTIONS:

Open the form and complete the front page as accurately and completely as possible. Describe each hazard you think exists in as much detail as you can. If the hazards described in your complaint are not all in the same area, please identify where each hazard can be found at the worksite. If there is any particular evidence that supports your suspicion that a hazard exists (for instance, a recent accident or physical symptoms of employees at your site) include the information in your description. If you need more space than is provided on the form, continue on any other sheet of paper.

After you have completed the form, return it to your local OSHA office.

NOTE: It is unlawful to make any false statement, representation or certification in any document filed pursuant to the Occupational Safety and Health Act of 1970. Violations can be punished by a fine of not more than $10,000. or by imprisonment of not more than six months, or by both. (Section 17(g))

Public reporting burden for this voluntary collection of information is estimated to vary from 15 to 25 minutes per response with an average of 17 minutes per response, including the time for reviewing instructions, searching existing data sources, gathering and maintaining the data needed, and completing and reviewing the collection of information. An Agency may not conduct or sponsor, and persons are not required to respond to the collection of information unless it displays a valid OMB Control Number. Send comment regarding this burden estimate or any other aspect of this collection of information, including suggestions for reducing this burden to the Directorate of Enforcement Programs, Department of Labor, Room N-3119, 200 Constitution Ave., NW, Washington, DC; 20210.

OMB Approval# 1218-0064; Expires: 05-31-2014

Do not send the completed form to this Office.

OSHA-7(Rev. 9/93)

FIGURE 2-5.

The OSHA complaint form can be completed online or on hard copy. It is available at http://www.osha.gov/oshforms/osha7.pdf.

U. S. Department of Labor
Occupational Safety and Health Administration

Notice of Alleged Safety or Health Hazards

Complaint Number	

Establishment Name			
Site Address			
	Site Phone	/	Site FAX
Mailing Address			
	Mail Phone		Mail FAX
Management Official		Telephone	
Type of Business			

HAZARD DESCRIPTION/LOCATION. Describe briefly the hazard(s) which you believe exist. Include the approximate number of employees exposed to or threatened by each hazard. Specify the particular building or worksite where the alleged violation exists.

Has this condition been brought to the attention of:	☐ Employer ☐ Other Government Agency(specify)
Please Indicate Your Desire:	☐ Do NOT reveal my name to my Employer ☐ My name may be revealed to the Employer
The Undersigned believes that a violation of an Occupational Safety or Health standard exists which is a job safety or health hazard at the establishment named on this form.	(Mark "X" in ONE box) ☐ Employee ☐ Federal Safety and Health Committee ☐ Representative of Employees ☐ Other (specify)

Complainant Name		Telephone	
Address(Street,City,State,Zip)			
Signature		Date	

If you are an authorized representative of employees affected by this complaint, please state the name of the organization that you represent and your title:

Organization Name: Your Title:

2

OSHA-7(Rev. 3/96)

FIGURE 2-5. *(Continued)*

■ Telephone: OSHA staff are available by telephone to discuss complaints and questions: 1-800-321-OSHA.

Employees are protected by a whistleblower law, which states that employers cannot punish employees for alerting OSHA to workplace hazards. *Employees cannot be fired, demoted, or harassed for filing a complaint with OSHA.*

Safety Practices Based on OSHA Standards

OSHA standards and related laws do not dictate daily operations. Instead, OSHA creates and enforces workplace standards and requires written workplace safety plans to improve workplace safety. Safety plans document best practices and SOPs that are provided by agencies and organizations with expertise in infection control as well as chemical and radiation safety. For example, OSHA does not prescribe the specifications of each type of personal protective equipment. Instead, OSHA requires that the equipment meet the standards of a recognized agency such as the **American National Standards Institute (ANSI)**. ANSI examines and endorses personal protective equipment such as goggles manufactured to its specifications, and because OSHA recognizes ANSI as an expert in this field, ANSI-approved goggles meet OSHA standards.

For facilities to be accredited, they must meet certain standards. For example, the Joint Commission requires that to receive its accreditation, institutions must have procedures, plans, and equipment that meet safety and infection control standards.

Table 2-4 ■ lists agencies, organizations, and nongovernmental organizations that provide information and standards for best practices in safety and infection control. These and others are discussed further in Chapters 3 through 7.

TABLE 2-4. Resources for Infection Control and Safety

Standards, Laws, Regulations

American National Standards Institute www.ansi.org

Clinical Laboratory Standards Institute www.clsi.org

Department of Energy www.doe.gov

Food and Drug Administration www.fda.gov

National Fire Protection Association www.nfpa.org

Nuclear Regulatory Commission www.nrc.gov

Occupational Safety and Health Administration www.osha.gov

Resources for Best Practices

American Chemical Society www.acs.org

American Conference of Governmental Industrial Hygienists www.acgih.org

Association for Professionals in Infection Control and Epidemiology www.apic.org

Centers for Disease Control and Prevention www.cdc.gov

National Institute for Occupational Safety and Health www.niosh.gov

Accrediting Body

Joint Commission www.jointcommission.org

Chapter Summary

- Agencies and laws help healthcare workers maintain a safe workplace.

- Governmental and nongovernmental organizations (NGOs) guide best practices in infection control as well as chemical and radiation safety.

- OSHA standards help protect employees from exposure to infectious, blood-borne, chemical, and radiation hazards.

- The OSHA Bloodborne Pathogens Standard is the primary standard guiding best practices in infection control.

- The OSHA Occupational Exposure to Hazardous Chemicals in Laboratories Standard is the primary standard guiding best practices in chemical safety.

- The OSHA Ionizing Radiation standard, the Department of Energy (DOE) Radiation Protection standard, and Nuclear Regulary Commission (NRC) Occupational Radiation Protection standards guide best practices in radiation safety.

- A written safety plan anchors each safety standard.

- The American National Standards Institute, the Association for Professionals in Infection Control and Epidemiology, the American Conference of Governmental Industrial Hygienists, the Centers for Disease Control and Prevention, and other agencies describe specific safety practices that are based on OSHA standards.

Application

Case Study 2-1: What Does OSHA Say about a Mandatory Flu Vaccine?

In April 2009, a novel H1N1 influenza A was identified, prompting the development and administration of vaccines to susceptible persons, including healthcare workers. A medical office assistant asked whether her employer can require employees to accept the flu shot. The employer is threatening employees with mandatory time off if they do not accept the flu shots.

Reference: Occupational Safety and Health Administration, Standard Interpretations. www .OSHA.gov

Questions:

1. Can the medical office require employees to accept the flu vaccine? Explain your answer.

2. How does this scenario change if the employee refuses the vaccine because she has severe reactions to flu vaccines?

Case Study 2-2: Contacting OSHA Is a Protected Right

A veteran clinic employee with many years of experience as an office assistant raised concerns about a new office procedure that required workers to remove protective caps from contaminated needles before putting the needles in sharps disposal containers. She felt that the new procedure exposed employees to injury and possible infection by blood-borne pathogens. Her employer did not take her complaints seriously. Alarmed at the potential danger, she filed a health hazard complaint with the Occupational Safety and

Health Administration. The complaint was investigated, and the employer was ordered to correct the procedure and was fined $26,000. After filing the complaint, the employee was fired. She challenged the termination. Her employer said that she did not handle the problem professionally because the actions embarrassed him and his practice.

Questions:

1. Did the employee act correctly in this situation? Explain.

2. Was the employer correct in firing the employee? Explain.

Assessment

Select the one best answer.

1. OSHA is a branch of the _____.
   a. Association of Professionals in Infection Control and Epidemiology
   b. Centers for Disease Control and Prevention
   c. U.S. Department of Labor
   d. National Institute of Occupational Safety and Health

2. Which standard specifically describes protection against transmission of HIV and hepatitis?
   a. Hazard Communication
   b. Bloodborne Pathogens
   c. Clinical Laboratory Improvement Amendments
   d. Occupational Exposure to Hazardous Chemicals in the Laboratory

3. A chemical hygiene plan is required by which standard?
   a. Hazard Communication
   b. Bloodborne Pathogens
   c. Clinical Laboratory Improvement Amendments
   d. Occupational Exposure to Hazardous Chemicals in the Laboratory Standard

4. Which organization regulates radiation in the workplace?
   a. NIOSH
   b. Nuclear Regulatory Commission
   c. U.S. Department of Labor
   d. CDC

5. An exposure control plan is a required component of which standard?
   a. Hazard Communication
   b. Bloodborne Pathogens
   c. Clinical Laboratory Improvement Amendments
   d. Occupational Exposure to Hazardous Chemicals in the Laboratory Standard

Resources

American Chemical Society www.acs.org
American Conference of Governmental Industrial Hygienists www.acgih.org
American National Standard Institute www.ansi.org

Association for Professionals in Infection Control and Epidemiology www.apic.org
Bureau of Labor Statistics www.bls.gov
Centers for Disease Control and Prevention www.cdc.gov
Clinical Laboratory Standards Institute www.clsi.org
Department of Energy www.doe.gov
Food and Drug Administration www.fda.gov
Joint Commission www.jointcommission.org
National Fire Protection Association www.nfpa.org
National Institute for Occupational Safety and Health www.niosh.gov
Nuclear Regulatory Commission www.nrc.gov
Occupational Safety and Health Administration www.osha.gov

PEARSON
myhealthprofessionskit™

Visit www.myhealthprofessionskit.com to access the interactive Companion Website for this textbook. Simply select "Basic Health Science" from the choice of disciplines. Find this book and log in using your user name and password to access additional learning tools.

CHAPTER 3

Infectious Diseases and Healthcare-Associated Infections

This chapter defines and illustrates infectious diseases and healthcare-associated infections (HAIs). The nature of infectious diseases, the importance of HAIs, and the main types of HAIs are described. Agents of biological terrorism are also discussed.

Objectives

After completing this chapter, the student will be able to:

- Define communicable disease and infectious disease.
- Know the types of microorganisms that cause infectious disease.
- Explain the chain of infection and how infectious diseases are transmitted.
- Describe the main types of healthcare-associated infections.
- Understand the problem of antibiotic resistance, such as methicillin-resistant *Staphylococcus aureus* (MRSA) and vancomycin-resistant enterococci (VRE).
- Identify the chief routes of healthcare-associated infection transmission.
- Name healthcare-associated infections associated with ambulatory care and other healthcare settings.
- Name the chief agents of biological terrorism.

Key Terms and Concepts

antibiotic resistance
bacteria
catheter-associated urinary tract
  infections (CAUTIs)
chain of infection

communicable disease
dialysis
fomite
fungi
healthcare-associated infection (HAI)

helminths

immune compromised

infectious disease

intravascular catheter–associated
  bloodstream infection

methicillin-resistant *Staphylococcus
  aureus* (MRSA)

mode of transmission

nosocomial infections

notifiable diseases

opportunist

pathogen

portal of entry

portal of exit

protozoa

reservoir

surgical site infections (SSI)

susceptible host

tissue graft

urinary tract infections (UTI)

vancomycin-resistant enterococci
  (VRE)

vector

ventilator-associated pneumonia
  (VAP)

virus

worms

Pathogenic Microorganisms

Each year, **infectious diseases** cause approximately 17 million deaths, one-third of all deaths worldwide. Of course, many more than 17 million fall ill each year, becoming disabled and missing education and work. Certain infections are especially contagious, harmful, or have no effective treatment (Appendix A). These infections, called **notifiable diseases**, must be reported to the Centers for Disease Control and Prevention (CDC) so that the incidence of these diseases can be carefully monitored.

Microorganisms that cause infectious disease are called **pathogens** or pathogenic microorganisms and include bacteria, viruses, fungi, protozoa, and worms (described in next section). Infectious diseases are described as **communicable diseases** and are capable of being transmitted directly from host to host. Tuberculosis, hepatitis B, influenza, HIV, and measles are communicable infectious diseases that are directly transmitted from person to person. Some infectious diseases are not transmitted directly from person to person; these infections require a carrier or **vector** to be transmitted to a host. For example, *Anopheles* mosquitoes transmit malaria; food contaminated with fecal matter transmits salmonellosis; raccoons, foxes, and bats transmit rabies. **Fomites** are inanimate objects that carry pathogens. These include skin cells and hair that individuals regularly shed, bedding, and other objects people touch. In healthcare settings, fomites can be any contaminated objects, for example, stethoscopes, catheters, needles, other medical instruments, and healthcare workers' clothing.

A **chain of infection** can be described for each pathogen. Breaking any link in this chain can control transmission of the pathogen. Figure 3-1 illustrates the components of a chain of infection. The pathogen here is *Staphylococcus aureus*, which is carried in the nasal passages of about 30% of the population and is a common skin contaminant. A strain of *S. aureus* is the cause of MRSA, a drug-resistant skin and tissue infection. In the healthcare workplace, the **reservoir** is usually infected patients. Some patients simply carry *S. aureus* in their noses, while others have infected wounds. The **portal of exit** describes how the pathogen leaves the reservoir. In this case, the pathogen can be expelled

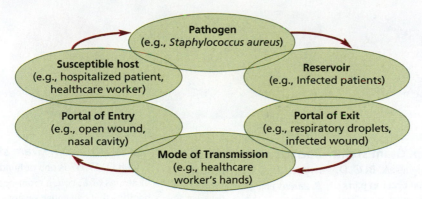

FIGURE 3-1.

Chain of infection. Each pathogen requires a susceptible host and access to a portal of entry, where the pathogen enters and begins an infection.

in respiratory droplets when sneezing and coughing; it can contaminate skin, or it can be found in the blood, pus, and debris of infected wounds. The **mode of transmission** describes how a pathogen is transferred to a new host. Here, hand contact is the mode of transmission. Healthcare workers can contaminate their hands with respiratory droplets or by touching material from infected wounds. The **portal of entry** is the means by which a pathogen enters the new host. *S. aureus* uses the nasal cavity or an open wound to gain access to a susceptible host. The **susceptible host** in healthcare settings can include another patient, a healthcare worker, or a patient's visitors. Susceptible hosts are plentiful in healthcare settings. Patients with open wounds, surgical wounds, weakened immune systems, underlying infections, HIV/AIDS, cancer, and malnutrition are all susceptible to infection.

Bacteria

Bacteria are single-celled microorganisms that are found in nearly every habitat, including the surfaces and interior of the human body. Bacteria exhibit great diversity, adapting well to varying food sources, absence or presence of oxygen, temperature and chemical extremes, even antibiotics. Most medically significant bacteria fall into two or three categories, based on the structure of their cell walls and their resulting staining properties (Figures 3-2 through 3-4). Bacteria are also described and classified by the shapes of their cells. A spherical cell is a coccus (plural, cocci). A chain of cocci is described as streptococci, a grape-bunch cluster is a staphylococcus, and a pair of cells is called diplococci. A rod-shaped cell is a bacillus (plural, bacilli), a curved rod is a vibrio, and a corkscrew-shaped cell is a spirochete.

Bacterial cell walls contain a unique complex sugar molecule called peptidoglycan. Gram-positive bacteria possess thick peptidoglycan walls, which permit them to retain the purple dye of the Gram stain. Some gram-positive pathogens produce endospores, structures resistant to extreme temperatures and dehydration. Special precautions such as autoclaving, incineration, or chemical treatments must be taken to eliminate these resistant forms. Endospore-producing gram-positive bacilli include various species that cause tetanus, botulism, anthrax, gangrene, and food poisoning. Gram-negative bacteria have cells with thinner peptidoglycan walls. Gram-negative cells are washed clear of

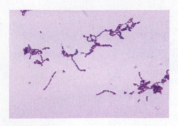

FIGURE 3-2.
Streptococcus **spp. Gram stain.**
Six groups are in this genus: A, B, C, D, F, and G. The cells often occur in pairs or chains. This gram-positive organism causes respiratory infections such as pneumonia and sinusitis, as well as bacteremia, otitis media, meningitis, peritonitis, and arthritis.

Source: Centers for Disease Control and Prevention. Public Health Image Library.

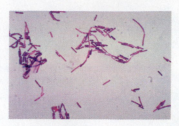

FIGURE 3-3.
Bacillus cereus **subsp.**
mycoides. **Gram stain.**
B. cereus is a gram-positive bacillus that is found in soil and causes food poisoning.

Source: Centers for Disease Control and Prevention. Public Health Image Library CDC/Dr. William A. Clark.

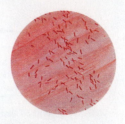

FIGURE 3-4.
Escherichia coli. **Gram stain.**
E. coli O157:H7 is one of hundreds of strains of *E. coli*, a gram-negative bacillus that can cause severe bloody diarrhea and abdominal cramps, and in some cases even death.

Source: Centers for Disease Control and Prevention. Public Health Image Library.

the Gram stain's purple dye and are stained pink in a subsequent step of the Gram stain process. A third group of bacteria is identified using a specially designed pink stain, the acid-fast stain. These bacteria include the bacilli *Mycobacterium tuberculosis* and *M. leprae*, the causes of tuberculosis and Hansen's disease (leprosy), respectively. Selected medically important bacterial pathogens as well as their associated diseases are listed in Table 3-1 ■.

Viruses

Viruses parasitize living cells, using their hosts' metabolic machinery to reproduce. Not considered a living organism, a **virus** consists of a nucleic acid wrapped in a protein coat, in some cases surrounded by a lipid envelope (Figure 3-5). Because viruses possess none of the conventional structures of cells, they depend entirely on cells for reproduction. In the course of reproducing, viruses damage cells in different ways: killing cells outright, altering cell structure and function, or transforming cells into tumors. Viruses infect specific host species and are adapted for certain tissues within the host. Thus the human influenza virus infects only human respiratory epithelium and not other species or other human tissues. Table 3-2 ■ lists selected viruses of medical importance and their associated diseases.

Fungi

Fungi are single-celled or multicelled microorganisms that absorb nutrients from the environment via filamentous structures called hyphae (Figure 3-6). Fungi, like animals and plants, consist of cells that are larger and more complex than bacterial cells. Most fungi cause no disease, playing the ecological role of decomposer. Those fungi that are pathogenic usually are **opportunists**, taking advantage of hosts with weakened immunity or damaged organs and tissues. Opportunistic fungal pathogens thrive in damaged or immune compromised human tissue (Table 3-3 ■).

TABLE 3-1. Selected Medically Important Bacteria

Bacteria	Disease(s)
Gram-Positive Bacteria	
MRSA (methicillin-resistant *Staphylococcus aureus*)	Antibiotic-resistant staphylococcal infections
Staphylococcus aureus	Staphylococcal infections, abscesses, osteomyelitis, food poisoning, pneumonia, toxic shock
Streptococcus pneumoniae ("pneumococcus")	Pneumonia
Streptococcus pyogenes	Pharyngitis, skin infections, otitis media, necrotizing fasciitis
Endospore-Forming Gram-Positive Bacteria	
Bacillus anthracis	Anthrax
Bacillus cereus (Figure 3-3)	Food poisoning
Clostridium botulinum	Botulism
Clostridium difficile ("C diff")	Colitis, diarrhea, sepsis
Clostridium perfringes	Gas gangrene
Clostridium tetani	Tetanus
Corynebacterium diphtheria	Diphtheria
Gram-Negative Bacteria	
Bordetella pertussis	Pertussis (whooping cough)
Borrelia burgdorferi	Lyme disease
Chlamydia trachomatis	Urethritis, pelvic inflammatory disease, trachoma, pneumonia
Escherichia coli (Figure 3-4)	Food poisoning, hemolytic uremia, urinary tract infections
Haemophilus influenzae	Meningitis, otitis media, pneumonia
Legionella pneumophila	Legionellosis
Listeria monocytogenes	Listeriosis
Neisseria gonorrhoeae ("gonococcus")	Gonorrhea
Neisseria meningitides ("meningococcus")	Meningococcal meningitis
Rickettsia rickettsii	Spotted fever rickettsiosis (Rocky Mountain spotted fever)

(Continued)

TABLE 3-1. *(Continued)*

Bacteria	Disease(s)
Salmonella typhi	Salmonellosis
Shigella flexneri	Dysentery
Treponema pallidum	Syphilis
VRE (vancomycin-resistant enterococci), usually *Enterococcus faecium* and some *Enterococcus faecalis*	Wound and bowel infections, urinary tract infections, sepsis, endocarditis, meningitis
Yersinia pestis	Plague
Acid-Fast Bacteria	
Mycobacterium leprae	Hansen's disease (leprosy)
Mycobacterium tuberculosis	Tuberculosis

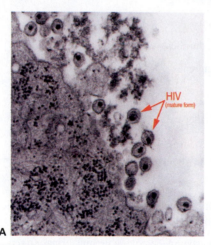
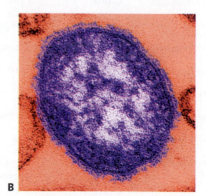

FIGURE 3-5.

Selected pathogenic viruses. (A) Human immunodeficiency virus (HIV). Transmission electron micrograph. Mature forms of HIV are indicated emerging from a human T cell (depicted in gray, lower left half of figure). (B) Measles virus. False color electron micrograph.

Source: Centers for Disease Control and Prevention. Public Health Image Library, (B) CDC/ Cynthia S. Goldsmith; William Bellini, Ph.D.

Protozoa

Protozoa inhabit any environment with enough moisture, including the human body. This group encompasses a wide variety of single-celled eukaryotic organisms, probably otherwise unrelated to each other (Figure 3-7). Protozoa exhibit animal-like traits such as locomotion and the need to ingest their nutrients. Like fungi, most protozoa cause no disease; however, included among protozoa are some of humanity's worst pathogens, including the causes of malaria, amebic dysentery, sleeping sickness, and opportunists that plague

TABLE 3-2. Selected Viruses of Medical Importance

Virus	Disease(s)
Cytomegalovirus	Chronic fatigue
Epstein-Barr	Mononucleosis
Hantavirus	Hantavirus pulmonary syndrome
Hepatitis A	Infectious hepatitis
Hepatitis B	Serum hepatitis
Hepatitis C	Hepatitis C
Herpes simplex type 1	Cold sores, skin sores
Herpes simplex type 2	Genital herpes
Human Immunodeficiency (Figure 3-5A)	HIV/AIDS
Influenza type A	Pandemic and epidemic flu
Influenza type B	Seasonal flu
Influenza type C	Seasonal flu
Lyssavirus (rabies virus)	Rabies
Morbillivirus (measles virus)	Rubeola (measles)
Rubellavirus	German measles (Figure 3-5B)
Rubulavirus (mumps virus)	Mumps
SARS-CoV (SARS-associated coronavirus)	Severe acute respiratory distress syndrome
Varicella zoster	Chickenpox

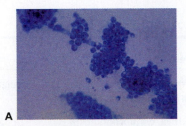
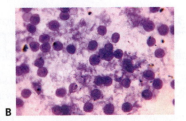

A   B

FIGURE 3-6.

Selected fungal pathogens. (A) *Candida albicans*. Methenamine silver stain. Pseudohyphae and true hyphae are visible. (B) *Pneumocystis jirovecii*. Toluidine blue stain. Smear of *P. jirovecii* concentrated from human lung.

Source: Centers for Disease Control and Prevention. Public Health Image Library (A) CDC/ Dr. Godon Roberstad, (B) CDC/ Lois Norman.

people with HIV/AIDS (Table 3-4 ■). As eukaryotes, both protozoa and worms resemble human cells in several ways. This poses some challenges for treatment and prevention. Even though the medications are effective, they can cause side effects, and it is difficult to develop vaccines for protozoa and worms.

TABLE 3-3. Selected Fungal Pathogens

Fungus	Disease(s)
Candida albicans (Figure 3-6A)	Candidiasis, urogenital yeast infections, oral thrush
Coccidioides immitis	Coccidiomycosis (valley fever or San Joaquin valley fever, respiratory disease); meningitis in patients with HIV/AIDS
Epidermophyton spp.	Athlete's foot, ringworm, jock itch
Histoplasma capsulatum	Histoplasmosis; chronic lung infection
Microsporum species	Athlete's foot, ringworm, jock itch
Pneumocystis jirovecii (Figure 3-6B)	Pneumonia in immune compromised, HIV/AIDS
Trichophyton species	Athlete's foot, ringworm, jock itch

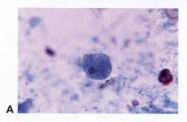 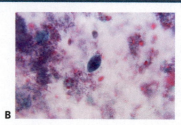

FIGURE 3-7.

Selected protozoan pathogens. (A) *Entamoeba histolytica*. Trichrome stain of liver aspirate. (B) *Giardia lamblia*. Trichrome stain revealing a *G. lamblia* cyst.

Source: Centers for Disease Control and Prevention. Public Health Image Library (A) CDC/ Dr. L.L.A. Moore, Jr., (B) CDC/Dr. Mae Melvin.

TABLE 3-4. Selected Pathogenic Protozoa

Protozoa	Disease(s)
Balantidium coli	Diarrhea, dysentery, balantidiasis; associated with malnutrition or HIV/AIDS
Cryptosporidium species	Diarrhea, cryptosporidiosis
Entamoeba histolytica (Figure 3-7A)	Dysentery, amebiasis
Giardia lamblia (Figure 3-7B)	Diarrhea, dysentery, giardiasis
Plasmodium species	Malaria

Worms

Among the most widespread pathogens, **worms**, or **helminths**, cause millions of infections and deaths worldwide each year. Worms are simple animals that exhibit a spectacular capacity for reproduction. Some worms possess complex organs and organ systems, while others with few organs have adopted entirely parasitic lives. Parasitic worms fall into two main categories, flatworms and roundworms, designations reflecting their overall body form (Figure 3-8). Parasitic worms range in size from a few millimeters to several meters. They may infest human blood, lymph, intestines, eyes, liver and bile ducts, and other sites (Table 3-5 ■).

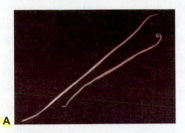
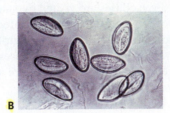
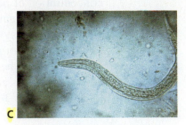

A   B   C

FIGURE 3-8.

Selected parasitic worms. (A) *Ascaris lumbricoides*. The larger of the two is the female of the species. The smaller male is on the right. Adult female worms can grow over 12 inches (30 cm) in length. (B) Eggs of *Enterobius vermicularis* mounted on cellulose tape. Eggs are deposited on perianal folds. Self-infection occurs by transferring infective eggs to the mouth with hands after scratching the perianal area. Person-to-person transmission can also occur through handling of contaminated clothes or bed linens. (C) Rhabditiform larva of the hookworm, *Necator americanus*. This is the worm's early, noninfectious immature stage. Larvae can become infective, that is, filariform stage, within feces and/or soil, and can then be passed to humans on contact.

Source: Centers for Disease Control and Prevention. Public Health Image Library.

TABLE 3-5. Selected Parasitic Worms

Worms	Disease(s)
Flatworms	
Clonorchis spp.	Liver flukes
Schistsoma spp.	Schistosomiasis (blood flukes)
Taenia, Echinococcus, Diphyllobothrium, Hymenolepsis spp.; tapeworms	Cysticercosis, neurocysticercosis, alveolar hydatid disease
Roundworms	
Ascaris lumbricoides (Figure 3-8A)	Intestinal infestation (ascariasis)
Brugia spp.	Filariasis, lymphatic infestation
Dracunculus medinensis	Guinea worm (subcutaneous filariasis)
Enterobius vermicularis (Figure 3-8B)	Pinworm (enterobiasis), large intestine infestation
Necator americanus (Figure 3-8C)	Hookworm, intestinal infestation
Onchocercus volvulus	Subcutaneous filariasis
Trichinella spp.	Trichinosis
Wuchereria bancrofti	Filariasis, lymphatic infestation

Healthcare-Associated Infections

Healthcare-associated infections (HAIs) are transmitted within healthcare facilities and are usually acquired from medical personnel or during medical procedures. Also commonly called **nosocomial infections**, their transmission is facilitated by the high concentration of patients, the use of invasive procedures, and close contact with medical personnel. Healthcare facilities are visited by many **immune compromised** patients, whose immune systems are weakened by viral infections, immunosuppressive therapy (for transplants or autoimmune diseases), poor nutrition, cancer, or HIV/AIDS. Special attention should be given to understanding the causes, transmission, and control of HAIs because patients and healthcare workers alike are at elevated risk for acquiring these infections (Table 3-6 ▪ and Appendix B).

TABLE 3-6. Selected HAIs

HAI	Transmission
Acinetobacter baumannii	Direct contact; respiratory infection associated with tracheostomy or ventilator, infects open wounds
Burkholderia cepacia	Direct contact; respiratory infection occurs with chronic lung disease and cystic fibrosis
Chickenpox (varicella)	Direct contact, respiratory droplets, and aerosolized virus from skin lesions
Clostridium difficile	Endospores and bacteria shed in feces, transmitted by contaminated hands and surfaces
Clostridium sordellii	Unknown; *C. sordellii* colonizes vagina in 29% of women after abortion; *C. sordellii* is detected in vaginal secretions of 5 to 10% of nonpregnant women
Ebola (viral hemorrhagic fever)	Contact with contaminated blood
Gastrointestinal (GI) infections	Contact with feces and contaminated materials
Hepatitis A	Contact with feces and contaminated materials
Hepatitis B	Contact with contaminated needles, contact with wounds and blood
Hepatitis C	Contact with contaminated needles, contact with wounds and blood
HIV/AIDS	Contact with contaminated needles, blood and body fluid, contact with open skin wound, eyes, mouth, nose
Influenza	Large respiratory droplets from coughing and sneezing
Intravascular catheter–associated bloodstream infections	Skin bacteria introduced to blood via intravenous catheter
MRSA: methicillin-resistant *Staphylococcus aureus*	Contact with skin, wounds, contaminated body fluids
Mumps	Respiratory droplets
Norovirus	Fecal-oral route

(Continued)

TABLE 3-6. *(Continued)*

HAI	Transmission
Pneumonia	Contact with contaminated hands, mainly associated with ventilators
SARS (Severe Acute Respiratory Syndrome)	Contact with respiratory droplets
Surgical site infection	Contact with skin and respiratory bacteria such as staphylococci or with GI bacteria
Tuberculosis	Airborne respiratory droplets from coughing, sneezing, talking, also during bronchoscopy and sputum collection
Urinary tract infections	Nearly all transmitted during catheterization
VISA: vancomycin-intermediate *Staphylococcus aureus*	Contact with skin, wounds, contaminated body fluids
VRE: vancomycin-resistant enterococci	Contact with contaminated skin

Several infectious diseases are especially associated with medical devices and procedures. **Urinary tract infections (UTIs)** account for 30% of HAIs acquired in hospitals. **Catheter-associated urinary tract infections (CAUTIs)** are named for UTIs that are associated with catheterization, which injures the urethral lining and introduces bacteria. Performing hand hygiene, disinfecting surfaces that come in contact with the patient, and using sterile catheters reduce the risk for CAUTIs.

Pneumonia is the second most common hospital-acquired infection, accounting for 15% of all infections and 27% of intensive care unit (ICU) infections. Most cases are associated with contaminated mechanical ventilators and related instruments and thus are named **VAPs (ventilator-associated pneumonias)**. A serious complication, VAP has a 20 to 33% mortality rate.

Surgical site infections (SSIs) account for 17% of all procedure-associated infections, affecting 1 to 3 of every 100 patients following surgery. Though surgery is relatively safe and most patients do not develop an SSI, with 46 million surgeries performed each year, this reflects a considerable number of cases.

Intravascular catheter–associated bloodstream infections are also relatively rare. But they are of great concern because peripheral intravenous catheters are commonly used, and these infections do cause considerable morbidity.

Dialysis and **tissue grafting** are also common procedures. Again, though they are relatively safe, the procedures put patients at risk for infections because these are invasive procedures that involve exchange of bodily fluid and tissue.

Antibiotic-Resistant Pathogens: MRSA and VRE

Antibiotic resistance has become a serious medical problem around the world. Several strains of pathogens have evolved resistance to drugs. In fact, certain strains of bacteria are resistant to multiple antibiotics, rendering them virtually impossible to treat.

Methicillin-resistant *Staphylococcus aureus* (MRSA) has occurred in hospitals for several years, and its incidence in the community has been increasing. A widespread gram-positive bacterium, *S. aureus* is carried in the nasal cavities of approximately 30% of people. About 1% of individuals carry MRSA. Around 7% of MRSA infections occur in people with no known contact with hospitals or hospital personnel. MRSA is primarily transmitted in healthcare settings in respiratory droplets and by contact. Chapter 4 discusses the precautions healthcare personnel need to take to prevent infections such as MRSA.

Enterococcus faecium and *E. faecalis* are gram-negative bacteria known as enterococci that normally live in the intestine and female genital tract. Usually they cause no problems, but on occasion, they cause infections in the blood, urinary tract, or wounds. When these bacteria enter the blood, they can cause meningitis and sepsis. Most infections occur in the hospital. Vancomycin resistance has developed in enterococci, but fortunately **vancomycin-resistant enterococci (VRE)** can be treated with other antibiotics. Precautions to take to prevent VRE and related infections are presented in Chapter 4.

TABLE 3-7. HAIs Associated with Different Healthcare Settings

Setting	HAI Risks
Ambulatory care	Occasional outbreaks documented for hepatitis A and C, tuberculosis, measles, rubella (obstetric outpatient setting), adenoviral conjunctivitis (ophthalmology outpatient setting), *Burkholderia* spp., and *Pseudomonas aeruginosa* (cystic fibrosis outpatient clinic)
Burn unit	High risk for patients with burns covering over 30% of body surface; *Staphylococcus aureus*, MRSA, VRE, *Candida* spp. aspergillosis, *Acinetobacter baumannii*, multidrug resistant *Pseudomonas aeruginosa*
Correctional facilities	Tuberculosis, scabies, meningococcal meningitis, pneumococcal pneumonia, gonorrhea, syphilis, HIV, hepatitis B, hepatitis C, hepatitis A, norovirus, MRSA
Home care	Catheter-associated bloodstream infections; other risks low due to reduced healthcare personnel contact, but risk exists for all respiratory and contact diseases
Intensive care unit	Setting for more than 26% of HAIs; VAP, venous catheter–associated infection, CAUTI, MRSA, VRE, *Candida* spp.
Long-term care	Influenza, rhinovirus, adenoviral conjunctivitis, norovirus, group A streptococci (*Streptococcus pyogenes*), pertussis, drug-resistant pneumococcal pneumonia, *Clostridium difficile*, MRSA, UTIs
Pediatrics	Pertussis, Respiratory Syncytial Virus (RSV) pneumonia, influenza, parainfluenza, adenovirus, measles, varicella, rotavirus
Shelters	Tuberculosis, scabies, meningococcal meningitis, pneumococcal pneumonia, gonorrhea, syphilis, HIV, hepatitis B, hepatitis C, hepatitis A, norovirus, MRSA

Source: Siegel JD, Rhinehart E, Jackson M, Chiarello L, and the Healthcare Infection Control Practices Advisory Committee, Centers for Disease Control and Prevention, 2007. Guideline for Isolation Precautions: Preventing Transmission of Infectious Agents in Healthcare Settings. Centers for Disease Control and Prevention.

> **WORDS OF WARNING!**
> ## Beware of the Pathogens at Work
> Pathogens in the healthcare workplace can infect humans and cause disease. These microorganisms are more virulent than those encountered in the community, can evade the immune system, and may be drug resistant. Some of these traits probably evolved within the healthcare environment. For example, antibiotic resistance evolved with modern widespread use of antibiotics, and antibiotic-resistant bacteria are much more prevalent within healthcare facilities than in the community. Suffice it to say that you'd rather not take workplace pathogens home with you to your family and friends. In Chapters 4 and 5, you'll learn more about controlling these pathogens.

Ambulatory Care–Associated Infections

In the ambulatory healthcare workplace, infections transmitted by respiratory droplets and hand contact are common. In general, these settings see occasional outbreaks of respiratory infections such as tuberculosis, measles, and influenza. Specific types of outpatient settings are associated with specific risks. For example, in obstetric outpatient settings, rubella has been documented, although rarely. Conjunctivitis caused by adenovirus, a respiratory virus, has been observed in ophthalmology outpatient clinics. At cystic fibrosis outpatient clinics, outbreaks of lung infections with *Burkholderia* spp. and *Pseudomonas aeruginosa* have been seen.

Other types of healthcare settings have unique HAI risks. For example, a greater incidence of SSIs and CAUTIs occur in hospitals than in ambulatory care, home care, or long-term care settings. Table 3-7 ■ describes the main risks associated with the various healthcare settings.

Agents of Bioterrorism

Healthcare facilities are expected to be among the first to detect a bioterrorism event. Bioterrorists could employ chemical, radiologic, or biologic agents. The biologic agents deployed may include the bacteria *Bacillus anthracis* (anthrax), *Yersinia pestis* (plague), *Clostridium botulinum* (botulism), or *Variola virus* (smallpox). Several other pathogens could be used, including the causes of tularemia, brucellosis, Q fever, viral hemorrhagic fevers, viral encephalitis, and staphylococcal enterotoxin B poisoning. The CDC maintains a comprehensive list and classification of biological agents (Box 3-1 ■).

BOX 3-1. Bioterrorism Agents

The CDC classifies bioterrorism agents into the following three categories:

CATEGORY A. Rarely seen in the United States, these high-priority agents include organisms that pose a risk to national security because they can be easily disseminated or transmitted from person to person, result in high mortality rates and have the potential for major public health impact, might cause public panic and social disruption, and require special action for public health preparedness. High-priority agents include the following:

- Anthrax (*Bacillus anthracis*)
- Botulism (*Clostridium botulinum* toxin)
- Plague (*Yersinia pestis*)

- Smallpox (variola major)
- Tularemia (*Francisella tularensis*)
- Viral hemorrhagic fevers (filoviruses [e.g., Ebola, Marburg] and arenaviruses [e.g., Lassa, Machupo])

CATEGORY B. Second highest priority agents include those that are moderately easy to disseminate, result in moderate morbidity rates and low mortality rates, and require specific enhancements of the CDC's diagnostic capacity and enhanced disease surveillance. These agents include the following:

- Brucellosis (*Brucella* species)
- Epsilon toxin of *Clostridium perfringens*
- Food safety threats (e.g., *Salmonella* species, *Escherichia coli* O157:H7, *Shigella*)
- Glanders (*Burkholderia mallei*)
- Melioidosis (*Burkholderia pseudomallei*)
- Psittacosis (*Chlamydia psittaci*)
- Q fever (*Coxiella burnetii*)
- Ricin toxin from *Ricinus communis* (castor beans)
- Staphylococcal enterotoxin B
- Typhus fever (*Rickettsia prowazekii*)
- Viral encephalitis (alphaviruses [e.g., Venezuelan equine encephalitis, eastern equine encephalitis, western equine encephalitis])
- Water safety threats (e.g., *Vibrio cholerae*, *Cryptosporidium parvum*)

CATEGORY C. Third highest priority agents include emerging pathogens that could be engineered for mass dissemination in the future because of availability, ease of production and dissemination, and potential for high morbidity and mortality rates and major health impact. Emerging pathogens include the following.

- Emerging infectious diseases such as Nipah virus and hantavirus

---

Source: Centers for Disease Control and Prevention www.cdc.gov

> **WORK SAFE!**
> ## Protection against the Unknown
> Does the next patient you're going to see carry a virus? Is she infected with a bacterium or a fungus? What part of his body is infected? Will viruses be in his blood or respiratory secretions? Is her skin contaminated with pathogens? You simply won't know whether the next person carries pathogens, is infected, or what kind of pathogen he or she may have. So what is your very best bet for protecting yourself and other patients? If you had to choose the single most important thing that you could do to prevent infections in this sort of scenario, what would you do? The answer is simple and highly effective. Performing hand hygiene regularly and correctly will control many infectious diseases. Good hand hygiene will be discussed in Chapter 4.

Your healthcare facility should have standard operating procedures for dealing with a bioterrorism event. While many precautions include those discussed in Chapters 4 and 5, additional steps may be necessary because of the nature of the biologic agents and the scale of the attack. Local Federal Bureau of Investigation (FBI) field offices provide guidelines to healthcare facilities for identifying terrorism events and directions for isolation, standard precautions, patient placement and transport, and cleaning and disinfection of equipment and the environment. The FBI also provides instructions on discharging patients, handling casualties, and postexposure prophylaxis for healthcare workers.

Chapter Summary

- Pathogenic microorganisms cause infectious diseases.
- To control infectious disease, the chain of infection must be broken.
- Healthcare-associated infections are hazards for patients and healthcare workers.
- Antibiotic-resistant bacteria are an emerging healthcare threat.
- Different HAIs are associated with different healthcare settings.
- A bioterrorism event may be first detected in healthcare facilities.

Application

Case Study 3-1: Break a Chain of Infection

Hepatitis B virus (HBV) infection broke out within an elder care facility affecting only patients with type 2 diabetes. Investigation found that the staff at the nursing home used a glucometer, a pen-like finger-stick device (Figure 3-9), to monitor the blood glucose of these patients. It was determined that the glucometer was not routinely cleaned between patients and therefore was occasionally contaminated with patient blood.

Questions:

1. Identify the links in this chain of infection:

   Pathogen
   Reservoir
   Portal of exit
   Mode of transmission
   Portal of entry
   Susceptible host

2. Explain how you can break this chain of infection.

Case Study 3-2: MRSA

It is important for workers to take precautions to prevent transmission of methicillin-resistant *Staphylococcus aureus* (MRSA), which occurs primarily in healthcare settings. MRSA is shed in blood, pus, and debris from MRSA-infected wounds. It can also colonize the nasal cavity. As a healthcare worker, you might be involved in direct patient care, or you might be serving patients another way in a clinic or office. Consider what you would do if one of your patients is diagnosed with MRSA.

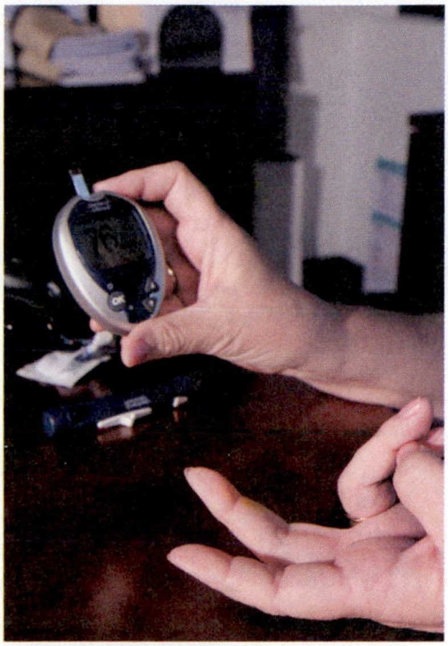

FIGURE 3-9.
Glucometer and finger-stick pen (glucolet).

Source: Centers for Disease Control and Prevention. Public Health Image Library CDC/Amanda Mills.

Questions:

1. Use what you have learned in this chapter to construct a possible chain of infection for this MRSA.

2. What do you think is the weakest link in the MRSA chain of infection? That is, explain what you think is the most effective way to prevent MRSA.

Assessment

Select the one best answer.

1. Each term is paired with a description. Which pair is incorrect?
   a. bacterium :: single celled microorganism
   b. fomite :: insect or another animal that transmits pathogens to humans
   c. virus :: intracellular parasite
   d. pathogen :: disease-causing microorganism
   e. opportunist :: microorganism that causes disease in weakened host

2. All of the following are composed of cells except _____.
   a. protozoa
   b. fungi
   c. roundworms
   d. viruses
   e. bacteria

3. Antibiotics are effective against only _____.
   a. protozoa
   b. fungi
   c. roundworms
   d. viruses
   e. bacteria

4. Which causes most of the healthcare-associated infections?
   a. surgical site infections
   b. catheter-associated infections
   c. ventilator-associated pneumonia
   d. urinary tract infections
   e. MRSA

5. What is the best way to prevent becoming infected with pathogens when working with a patient who has an infected wound?
   a. vaccination
   b. take antibiotics
   c. wear gloves and perform hand hygiene
   d. wear a face mask
   e. wear a sterile gown

Resources

American Society for Microbiology www.asm.org

Centers for Disease Control and Prevention www.cdc.gov

Siegel JD, Rhinehart E, Jackson M, Chiarello L, and the Healthcare Infection Control Practices Advisory Committee, Centers for Disease Control and Prevention. 2007. *Guideline for Isolation Precautions: Preventing Transmission of Infectious Agents in Healthcare Settings.* Centers for Disease Control and Prevention.

World Health Organization www.who.org

PEARSON
myhealthprofessionskit™

Visit www.myhealthprofessionskit.com to access the interactive Companion Website for this textbook. Simply select "Basic Health Science" from the choice of disciplines. Find this book and log in using your user name and password to access additional learning tools.

CHAPTER 4

Controlling Healthcare-Associated Infections

This chapter describes and illustrates methods for controlling healthcare-associated (nosocomial) infections.

Objectives

After completing this chapter, the student will be able to:

- Describe effective hand hygiene.
- Describe standard precautions and transmission-based precautions.
- Describe appropriate use of personal protective equipment (PPE) for infection control.
- Explain procedures for effective environmental hygiene.
- Describe the role of vaccination in infection control.

Key Terms and Concepts

airborne precautions
airborne infection isolation room
alcohol
antibodies
antigens
chlorhexidine gluconate
contact precautions
droplet precautions
ethanol
hand hygiene
iodine
iodophor
isopropyl alcohol

lymphocytes
n-propanol
personal protective equipment
polaxamer
povidone
resident flora
respiratory and cough etiquette
standard precautions
transient flora
transmission-based precautions
universal precautions
vaccination

Infection Control in the Workplace

Precautions significantly reduce the risk for transmitting healthcare-associated infections (HAIs). As discussed in Chapter 1, infection control in the healthcare workplace encompasses engineering controls, safe work practices, administrative controls, and personal protective equipment. Many situations call for some combination of these controls. This chapter discusses specific examples and applications of each of these controls, in both ambulatory and hospital settings.

Hand Hygiene

Microorganisms normally associated with the body are called **resident flora**. The skin's resident flora occupies the deeper layers of the epidermis. The superficial epidermis layer hosts **transient flora**, microorganisms that associate temporarily with the skin. Transient flora is acquired by contact from the environment and causes many infections transmitted by the hands. Therefore, direct and indirect contact with patients requires **hand hygiene** methods that reduce transient flora. However, the deeper resident flora also must be reduced when performing invasive procedures and surgery. This section describes hand hygiene for both scenarios.

The World Health Organization (WHO) and the Centers for Disease Control and Prevention (CDC) each publishes extensive reviews of hand hygiene, including the science underlying its practice, methods and antiseptic agents, and research on compliance and efficacy. The practice of hand hygiene begins with the question "*When* should I wash my hands?" WHO and CDC summarize the answer in "My five moments for hand hygiene" (Table 4-1 ■). One must practice hand hygiene before touching a patient and performing clean or aseptic procedures, and after a potential exposure and touching a patient or the patient's surroundings. Remember that microorganisms likely contaminate patient bedding, clothes, and nearby surfaces.

Having answered "When should I wash my hands?" the next question is "*How* do I wash my hands?" The choice of antiseptic agent and hygiene method depends on the situation and the types of potential pathogens. Consider the types of antiseptic agents available for hand hygiene. Each agent possesses properties that suit it for certain pathogens (Table 4-2 ■) and applications (Table 4-3 ■). Ordinary hand soap and tap water only moderately reduce transient flora on the hands. Plain soap has minimal antimicrobial activity. Moreover, studies have linked contaminated tap water to nosocomial infections. Thus it is recommended that healthcare workers use soaps and products that contain antimicrobial agents.

Alcohols (**ethanol, isopropyl alcohol, n-propanol**) in solution of 60 to 70% exhibit excellent antimicrobial activity against gram-positive bacteria, gram-negative bacteria, mycobacteria, fungi, and many enveloped viruses. Alcohols cannot be used to control endospores, protozoa cysts, or some nonenveloped viruses. Many antimicrobial soaps and antiseptics contain alcohol and are commonly dispensed in gels and foams for hand-rubbing (not hand washing). When hand-rubbing, the alcohol solution is rubbed on the hands without water and allowed to *air dry*. Alcohols evaporate quickly, leaving no residual antimicrobial activity on the surface. However, alcohols are poor cleaning agents and should not be used for cleaning

TABLE 4-1. My Five Moments for Hand Hygiene

Moment	Routes of Hand Transmission	Prevented Negative Outcome
1. Before touching a patient	From: Any surface in the healthcare area To: Any surface in the patient zone	Patient colonization with healthcare microorganisms; rarely exogenous infection
2. Before clean/aseptic procedure	From: Any other surface To: Critical site with infectious risk for the patient	Patient endogenous infection; exceptionally exogenous infection
3. After body fluid exposure risk	From: Critical site with body fluid exposure risk or critical site with infectious risk To: Any other surface	Healthcare worker infection
4. After touching a patient	From: Any surface in the patient zone To: Any surface in the healthcare area	Healthcare worker colonization; environmental contamination
5. After touching patient surroundings	From: Any surface in the patient zone without touching the patient To: Any surface in the healthcare area	Healthcare worker cross-colonization; environmental contamination

Source: Advisory Committee and the HICPAC/SHEA/APIC/IDSA Hand Hygiene Task Force. 2002, October 25. *Guideline for Hand Hygiene in Healthcare Settings Recommendations of the Healthcare Infection Control Practices*. Centers for Disease Control and Prevention, MMWR, Recommendations and Reports Vol. 51.

TABLE 4-2. Antimicrobial Activity of Selected Hand Hygiene Antiseptics

+++ = highly effective
++ = effective
+ = somewhat effective
− = ineffective

Antiseptics	Gram-Positive Bacteria	Gram-Negative Bacteria	Viruses, Enveloped	Viruses, Nonenveloped	Mycobacteria	Fungi	Endospores
Alcohols	+++	+++	+++	++	+++	+++	—
Chlorhexidine gluconate	+++	++	++	+	+	+	—
Iodophors	+++	+++	++	++	++	++	+/−*

*In concentrations used in antiseptics, iodophors are not sporocidal.

Source: WHO Guidelines on Hand Hygiene in Healthcare. 2009. World Health Organization www.who.org

TABLE 4-3. Parameters and Applications of Selected Hand Hygiene Antiseptics

Antiseptics	Concentration, %	Speed of Action	Residual Activity	Use
Alcohols	60 to 70 %	Fast	No	As component of gels and foams; hand-rubbing before and after patient contact
Chlorhexidine gluconate	0.5 to 4 %	Intermediate	Yes	As component of disinfectant; 0.5 to 1% solutions for hand washing, 2 to 4 % for surgical scrub
Iodophors	0.5 to 10 %	Intermediate	+/-*	Hand washing and antiseptic for patient skin

*Evidence for iodophor residual activity is contradictory and depends on formulations, use, and concentrations.

Source: *WHO Guidelines on Hand Hygiene in Healthcare*. 2009. World Health Organization www.who.org

visibly soiled hands. Overall, alcohols are best used in hand-rub gels and foams, and are considered the gold standard for protecting patients from nosocomial infections transmitted by healthcare workers' hands. In the clinic or healthcare provider's office, healthcare workers and patients should have access to alcohol hand-rub dispensers at the reception desk and on walls inside examination and treatment rooms as well as bathrooms.

Chlorhexidine gluconate acts more slowly than alcohols but remains on the hands longer with residual antimicrobial activity. Chlorhexidine plus hand hygiene products in low concentrations are more effective than plain soaps for hand hygiene. Solutions with higher concentrations are used for surgical scrubbing. Chlorhexidine is effective for gram-positive bacteria, fungi, enveloped viruses; it is somewhat less effective for gram-negative bacteria; it is not effective for mycobacteria, endospores, and nonenveloped viruses. At outpatient clinics and healthcare providers' offices, antimicrobial soap dispensers often contain alcohol-based soaps and hand-rubs, and do not contain soaps with chlorhexidine gluconate.

Iodine and **iodophors** (**povidone** and **polaxamers**) are effective for antiseptic hand hygiene. Iodine in these solutions controls gram-positive bacteria, gram-negative bacteria, mycobacteria, fungi, and viruses, but they will not inactivate endospores. These are not often used in soap dispensers.

Other antimicrobial agents have been used in the past for hand hygiene but at this time are not recommended for hand hygiene because the U.S. Food and Drug Administration (FDA) has insufficient data to support their safety and efficacy. These agents include triclosan, quaternary ammonium compounds (benzalkonium chloride), chloroxylenol, and hexachlorophene.

Three methods for hand hygiene are described in the following sections. In some cases, hand washing or hand-rubbing are appropriate; however, preparing for invasive or surgical methods requires scrubbing.

Alcohol-Based Rubs

Use before and after routine contact with patients.

1. If hands are visibly soiled, wash hands with soap and water and dry before proceeding. The hands should be visibly clean and free of debris, dirt, excess oil, and organic material so that the alcohol can contact the skin and inactivate microorganisms (Figure 4-1).

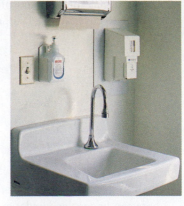

FIGURE 4-1.
Wash visibly soiled hands.

2. Apply a generous palmful of alcohol-hand-rub. The hand-rub may be a foam, lotion, or liquid. Cover all surfaces of the hands (Figure 4-2).
3. Rub all surfaces of hands, between fingers, and under and around nails until dry. At this point, hands are considered clean unless they touch a surface.

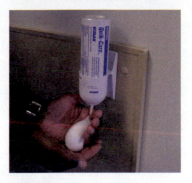

FIGURE 4-2.
Apply alcohol-based hand-rub.

Soap (Antimicrobial or Regular Soap) and Water

Use if hands are visibly soiled, skin is sensitive to alcohol rubs, or alcohol-based antiseptics are not readily available.

1. Wet hands with water. Water helps soap coat hand surfaces and helps inactivate microorganisms (Figure 4-3).

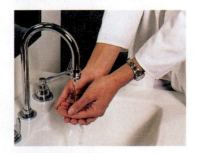

FIGURE 4-3.
Wet hands with water.

2. Apply a generous amount of soap to wet hands, enough to cover all hand surfaces (Figure 4-4).

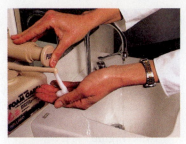

FIGURE 4-4.
Apply soap to wet hands.

3. Rub soapy water on all surfaces of hands, between fingers, and under and around nails. Rub vigorously and use friction to work soapy water on surfaces. Note that fingers should point down to drain microorganisms from the hands into the sink and to prevent contaminating hands and arms. Clean, running water should be used when rinsing so that microorganisms are washed from hand surfaces. Water temperature is not important, but hot water should be avoided because it increases risk for skin injury and infection or dermatitis (Figure 4-5).

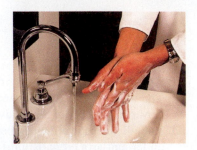

FIGURE 4-5.
Rub hands with soapy water.

4. Dry hands thoroughly with clean paper towels, and do not touch sink, clothes, or other objects to avoid contaminating the hands. Never reuse or share towels. At this point, hands are considered clean. To avoid contaminating the hands, turn off the water while holding a clean paper towel (Figure 4-6).

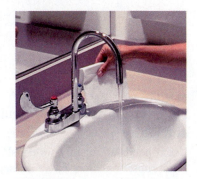

FIGURE 4-6.
Dry hands with paper towels.

Surgical Preparation

1. Remove jewelry and wrist watches before beginning. Artificial nails are prohibited.
2. Visibly soiled hands should be washed with plain soap and water before continuing. Remove debris from underneath fingernails using a nail cleaner, preferably under running water.
3. Do not wash with brushes because these cause abrasions.
4. Before putting on sterile gloves, wash with either an antimicrobial soap or alcohol-based hand-rub, preferably with an antimicrobial with residual activity, such as chlorhexidine gluconate.
5. If using an antimicrobial soap, wash hands and forearms for 2 to 5 minutes.
6. If using an alcohol-based hand-rub with sustained activity, follow the manufacturer's instructions for application times. Apply the product to dry hands only.
7. If using an alcohol-based hand-rub, use sufficient product to keep hands and forearms wet with the hand-rub throughout the surgical hand preparation procedure.
8. After application, dry hands and forearms thoroughly before putting on sterile gloves.

Figure 4-7 illustrates guidelines from the World Health Organization (WHO) for surgical hand preparation.

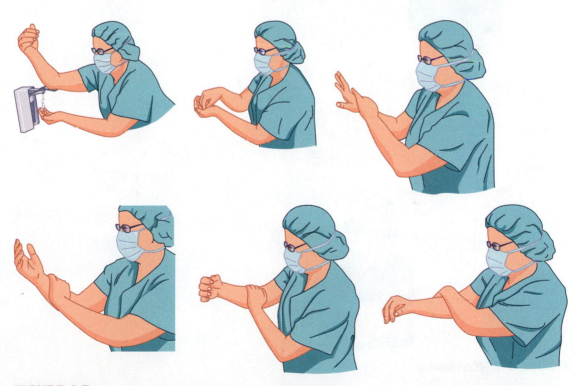

FIGURE 4-7.
Alcohol surgical scrub method.
Source: WHO Guidelines on Hand Hygiene in Health Care. World Health Organization. 2009.

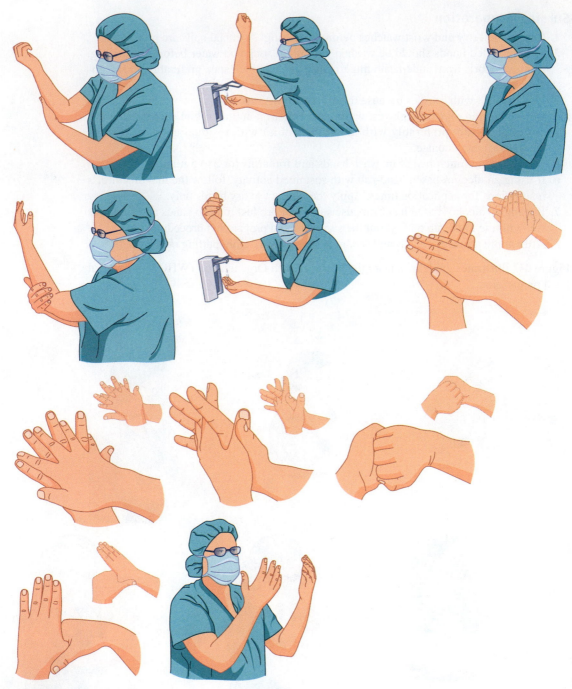

FIGURE 4-7. *(Continued)*

Standard Precautions

Standard precautions are applied when working with all patients, under all circumstances, whether or not patients are known to be infected. Standard precautions are intended to protect patients from infections transmitted by healthcare workers, and are based on the idea that blood, body fluids, skin wounds, and mucous membranes may contain pathogenic microorganisms. The components of standard precautions include hand hygiene; use of gloves, gown, mask, eye protection, or face shield; safe injection practices; and disinfection and safe handling of equipment that may have become contaminated (Table 4-4 ■). Three major practices have been added recently to standard precautions: respiratory hygiene and cough etiquette, safe injection practices, and use of masks for insertion of catheters and lumbar puncture procedures.

Universal precautions include the elements of standard precautions and were first developed to protect healthcare workers from hazards associated with blood-borne pathogens such as HIV and hepatitis B. Universal precautions are discussed in detail in Chapter 5.

TABLE 4-4. Recommendations for Application of Standard Precautions for the Care of All Patients in All Healthcare Settings

Component	Recommendations
Hand hygiene	After touching blood, body fluids, secretions, excretions, contaminated items; immediately after removing gloves; between patient contacts
Gloves	For touching blood, body fluids, secretions, excretions, contaminated items; for touching mucous membranes and nonintact skin
Gown	During procedures and patient-care activities when contact of clothing or exposed skin with blood, body fluids, secretions, and excretions is anticipated
Mask, eye protection (goggles), face shield	During procedures and patient-care activities likely to generate splashes or sprays of blood, body fluids, or secretions, especially suctioning, endotracheal intubation
Mask for catheter insertion or lumbar puncture	These procedures are likely to generate splashes or sprays of blood, body fluids, or secretions
Soiled patient-care equipment	Handle in a manner that prevents transfer of microorganisms to others and to the environment; wear gloves if equipment is visibly contaminated; perform hand hygiene
Environmental control	Develop procedures for routine care, cleaning, and disinfection of environmental surfaces, especially frequently touched surfaces in patient-care areas
Textiles and laundry	Handle in a manner that prevents transfer of microorganisms to others and to the environment
Safe injection practices, needles, and other sharps	Do not recap, bend, break, or hand-manipulate used needles; if recapping is required, use a one-handed scoop technique only; use safety features when available; place used sharps in puncture-resistant container

(Continued)

TABLE 4-4. *(Continued)*

Component	Recommendations
Patient resuscitation	Use mouthpiece, resuscitation bag, or other ventilation devices to prevent contact with mouth and oral secretions
Patient placement	Prioritize for single-patient room if patient is at increased risk of transmission, is likely to contaminate the environment, does not maintain appropriate hygiene, or is at increased risk of acquiring infection or developing an adverse outcome following infection
Respiratory hygiene and cough etiquette	Instruct symptomatic persons to cover mouth and nose when sneezing or coughing; use tissues and dispose in no-touch receptacle; observe hand hygiene after soiling of hands with respiratory secretions; wear surgical mask if tolerated; or maintain spatial separation, greater than 3 feet if possible

Source: Siegel JD, Rhinehart E, Jackson M, Chiarello L, and the Healthcare Infection Control Practices Advisory Committee. 2007. *Guideline for Isolation Precautions: Preventing Transmission of Infectious Agents in Healthcare Settings*. Centers for Disease Control and Prevention.

Transmission-Based Precautions

Sometimes standard precautions alone cannot block transmission of an infectious disease, especially if the disease can be transmitted in more than one way. In that case, a more focused approach called **transmission-based precautions** supplements standard precautions. Transmission-based precautions take into consideration the specific routes of transmission associated with specific infectious diseases and thus include the following three types of precautions: contact precautions, droplet precautions, and airborne precautions.

Contact Precautions

Contact precautions prevent contamination by pathogens that can be transmitted via direct or indirect contact. These precautions apply when patients are infected with antibiotic-resistant bacteria or if patients have wound drainage, diarrhea, or fecal incontinence. Numerous infections may be transmitted via contact, including methicillin-resistant *Staphylococcus aureus* (MRSA), vancomycin-resistant enterococci (VRE), *Clostridium difficile*, rotavirus, hepatitis A, herpes simplex, varicella zoster (shingles), impetigo, pediculosis (head lice), polio, *Burkholderia cepacia*, and streptococcal and staphylococcal skin infections. Patients should be housed singly or if in shared rooms, should be spaced three or more feet away from other patients. Healthcare workers should wear gloves, masks, and gowns when entering a patient's room and should remove these items before leaving the room.

Droplet Precautions

Droplet precautions prevent transmission of pathogens via respiratory droplets. These pathogens remain viable and infectious in the air over short distances, often less than six feet. Pathogens transmitted by droplets include *B. pertussis* (whooping cough), influenza virus (flu), adenovirus (respiratory infections and colds), rhinovirus (colds), *Neisseria meningitides* (meningitis), and group A streptococcus (ear, throat, and lung infections). As with contact precautions, patients should be housed singly or if in shared rooms, should be spaced three or more feet away from other patients. If a curtain is available between beds, it should be closed to control the spread of respiratory droplets between the beds. Every healthcare worker should wear a mask when entering the patient's room and remove it when leaving the room. If the patient must be moved from the room to another area, the patient should wear a mask during transport. Healthcare workers should advise the patient to practice respiratory and cough etiquette.

Workers should also practice **respiratory and cough etiquette** to reduce the transmission of infectious respiratory droplets. Patients and healthcare workers should cough or sneeze into the corner of their elbow, not into their hands. Used tissues should be disposed of, and hand hygiene should be performed after using tissues, coughing, or sneezing. If he or she is coughing, the patient should wear a mask.

Airborne Precautions

Airborne precautions prevent transmission of pathogens in small respiratory droplets that remain airborne, viable, and infectious over long distances. Such pathogens include rubeola virus (measles), *Mycobacterium tuberculosis* (tuberculosis), and varicella virus (chicken pox and shingles). In these cases, patients should be housed singly in **airborne infection isolation rooms** (AII), which are designed to contain airborne pathogens. These rooms have negative air pressure, which keeps room air from escaping to the surroundings. Room air should ventilate directly outside of the building or be filtered if it is returned to the room. Patients with active tuberculosis should be housed in AII rooms. Healthcare workers with close patient contact should wear respiratory protection. Some states require the use of AII rooms and respirators in healthcare facilities that treat tuberculosis. In addition, healthcare workers caring for patients with airborne diseases should be vaccinated if a vaccine is available for those specific diseases. Nonimmune workers should not care for these patients.

Ambulatory Care and Other Outpatient Settings

Healthcare workers should be prepared to employ infection control measures wherever they encounter patients. Such settings include ambulatory care, home care, and long-term care facilities.

Ambulatory Care

Most healthcare takes place outside hospitals in a variety of ambulatory care facilities and community clinics. Ambulatory care services are diverse, and each setting poses different risks. Ambulatory healthcare settings include outpatient surgery, urgent care, dialysis centers, ophthalmology clinics, and public health clinics. Many infectious diseases in these settings are transmitted by respiratory droplets, contact, contaminated devices, multiuse vials, or intravenous (IV) solutions. Therefore, infection control relies on good hand hygiene, respiratory and cough etiquette, and maintenance of clean equipment. These items can control many infectious diseases. Employers should post

WORDS OF WARNING!
Precautions for Tuberculosis

How should a facility prepare for working with tuberculosis patients? Tuberculosis (TB) is an airborne respiratory disease caused by the acid-fast bacillus *Mycobacterium tuberculosis*.

Therefore TB requires airborne transmission precautions and airborne infection isolation (AII) rooms. The CDC has developed three levels of precautions for TB.

I. **Administrative Controls.** This is the most important control for TB in a hospital because it affects the most people. The aim is to reduce the risk of transmission of TB from patients with active TB to uninfected persons. Managers must assign responsibility for TB infection control and must conduct a TB risk assessment for the facility. The TB infection control plan should describe detection, airborne precautions, and treatment of infected persons. Laboratory testing must be performed and reported rapidly and efficiently to the responsible physicians. Managers must ensure proper cleaning and sterilization or disinfection of potentially contaminated equipment (e.g., bronchoscopes, endoscopes) and train workers regarding TB prevention, transmission, and symptoms. Regular screening must be available for all workers at risk for TB disease or who might be exposed to *M. tuberculosis*. All occurrences of TB at the site must be investigated. The facility should use signs promoting respiratory hygiene and cough etiquette.

II. **Environmental Controls.** The next most important control is environmental controls to prevent the spread and reduce the concentration of infectious droplets in the air. These include the use of local exhaust ventilation (hoods, tents, or booths) in TB patient rooms and general ventilation to dilute and remove contaminated air in the facility. Negative pressure airflow should be used to prevent contamination of air in areas adjacent to the source (airborne infection isolation [AII] rooms). Air should be cleaned using high efficiency particulate air (HEPA) filtration, or ultraviolet germicidal irradiation.

III. **Protective Respiratory Equipment.** Protective respiratory equipment may be necessary when administrative and environmental controls are not adequate. Aerosolized infectious particles may be generated during surgical procedures and in other situations, posing a high risk of exposure to *M. tuberculosis*. A written formal respiratory protection program should describe training on proper use of respiratory protection. Patients and workers should be trained on respiratory hygiene and cough etiquette.

Source: Centers for Disease Control and Prevention

signs in suitable locations promoting and illustrating hand hygiene as well as respiratory and cough etiquette. Employers should also make available antiseptic handrub dispensers to encourage hand hygiene. Employees must adhere to safe injection practices as well as employer and manufacturer procedures for disinfecting medical equipment.

More vigilance is needed to control respiratory diseases targeted by airborne precautions: *M. tuberculosis*, varicella zoster virus, and rubeola virus (measles). As soon as infected patients are identified, they should be directed to use separate waiting areas to isolate them from other patients. Infected patients should be instructed to use respiratory and cough etiquette, and if coughing, they should wear a mask.

Ambulatory healthcare workers should be aware that MRSA can be transmitted outside of hospitals. The incidence of community-acquired MRSA (CA-MRSA) has been increasing, and there are reports of healthcare workers becoming infected with CA-MRSA at their workplace. This reinforces the importance of practicing hand hygiene in the workplace.

Home Care

Home healthcare includes many services, such as assistance with activities of daily living, ambulatory peritoneal dialysis, infusion therapy, and wound care. The risks for infection are reduced in these settings because usually only one patient receives care in each setting, one or very few healthcare workers are involved, and few medical devices and solutions are shared with other patients. The chief reservoirs of infection are the infected healthcare worker, the infected patient, and contaminated equipment. Common infections transmitted to the patient include catheter-associated bloodstream infections and respiratory infections. Home healthcare workers are at risk for acquiring respiratory infections such as influenza, chickenpox, and tuberculosis, as well as skin contact diseases such as scabies and impetigo. Employees should adhere to all standard precautions and employer guidelines.

Long-Term Care

Unlike the typical outpatient clinic and the hospital, a long-term care facility houses a community of residents who spend much time together, often in close contact. Controlling respiratory and contact infections is difficult when residents regularly share eating and recreational areas. Most experts agree that residents gain many mental health benefits from regular social contact with peers. However, residents of these facilities are often immunocompromised and vulnerable to infection, so it is important to monitor and detect diseases early so that residents can receive treatment and be isolated if necessary. In addition, long-term care residents often make frequent trips to hospitals or other healthcare facilities, where they are exposed to infectious agents, become colonized, and carry the agents back to the long-term care facility. Plus, healthcare staff can transmit infectious diseases to these vulnerable residents. Thus it is necessary to strictly adhere to standard precautions and transmission-based precautions when indicated.

Personal Protective Equipment

Whether healthcare workers are employed in ambulatory or inpatient settings, **personal protective equipment** (PPE) should be used if contact with patient blood or body fluids is anticipated or likely. The barrier provided by PPE improves infection control considerably, but to be effective, PPE must be used correctly. For example, PPE must be put on and removed in such a way as to prevent contamination. Also, to prevent spreading pathogens to adjacent areas or other patients, PPE must be removed when leaving the patient area. PPE includes gloves, isolation gowns, masks, eye protection, and at times respirators.

Gloves

Disposable latex or nitrile gloves provide effective barriers during contact with blood, body fluids, wounds, or other possible sources of pathogens (Box 4-1 ■). To be effective, gloves must be donned, removed, and disposed of correctly. Figure 4-8 describes the method for donning and removing disposable latex or nitrile gloves. Figure 4-9 describes the method for donning and removing sterile gloves, such as those used during surgery. Gloves must never be reused, washed, or worn while caring for more than one patient. If gloves become damaged or contaminated during use, they must be discarded and replaced.

BOX 4-1. World Health Organization Guidelines on Hand Hygiene in Healthcare: Situations Requiring and not Requiring Glove Use

STERILE GLOVES INDICATED Any surgical procedure; vaginal childbirth; invasive radiological procedures; performing vascular access and procedures (central lines); preparing total parenteral nutrition and chemotherapeutic agents

EXAMINATION (NON-STERILE) GLOVES INDICATED IN CLINICAL SITUATIONS *Potential for touching blood, body fluids, secretions, excretions, and items visibly soiled by body fluids*

Direct patient exposure: Contact with blood; contact with mucous membrane and with nonintact skin; potential presence of highly infectious and dangerous organisms; epidemic or emergency situations; inserting and removing IV lines; drawing blood; giving subcutaneous and intramuscular injections; discontinuing of venous line; performing pelvic and vaginal examination; suctioning non-closed systems of endotracheal tubes.

Indirect patient exposure: Emptying emesis basins; handling and cleaning instruments; handling waste; cleaning up spills of body fluids

GLOVES NOT INDICATED (EXCEPT FOR CONTACT PRECAUTIONS) *No potential for exposure to blood or body fluids, or contaminated environment*

Direct patient exposure: Taking blood pressure, temperature, and pulse; bathing and dressing a patient with no potential for exposure to infectious material; transporting a patient with no potential for exposure to infectious material

Indirect patient contact: Using the telephone; writing in the patient chart; giving oral medications; distributing or collecting patient dietary trays; removing and replacing linens for patient bed if not visibly soiled; moving patient furniture; placing noninvasive ventilation equipment and nasal oxygen cannula

Gowns

Isolation gowns prevent contamination of clothes and skin during procedures that expose healthcare workers to blood, body fluids, or urine and fecal material, or when the patient produces uncontained secretions, as occur with incontinence or profuse bleeding. To prevent contamination of hands, hand hygiene must be performed before and immediately after gown use. In addition, care must be taken when donning and removing gowns to prevent contamination, especially when using sterile gowns for surgery (Figure 4-10). Gowns must be removed and disposed of when leaving the patient area; gowns must never be reused. Note that clinical laboratory coats and jackets worn for identification as a healthcare worker or for comfort are not considered PPE.

FIGURE 4-8.

Donning and removing disposable gloves.

1. Before donning gloves, wash hands with soap and water or an alcohol-based hand-rub. Use foot pedal if available to operate the faucet without contaminating hands.

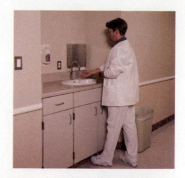

2. Alcohol-based hand-rubs require no water.

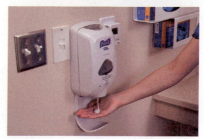

3. Select correct size gloves. Small gloves may tear, and large gloves may slip off or bunch up and tear.

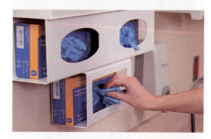

4. Grasp the base of one glove, holding its inner surface, and pull it over your hand.

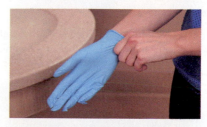

5. Pull on the other glove, taking care not to stretch or tear the gloves.

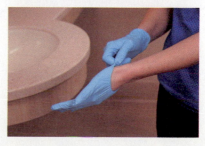

6. To remove gloves, begin by grasping one glove near the wrist with the other gloved hand. Avoid touching the outside surfaces of gloves with ungloved hands.

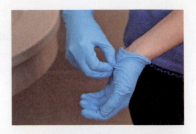

7. With the gloved hand, peel the glove off the other hand, turning it inside out.

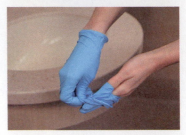

8. Enclose the glove just removed in the palm of the gloved hand.

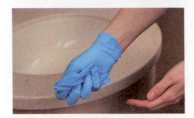

9. Remove the other glove by first sliding fingers between the glove and the wrist. This exposes the hand to the clean inner surface of the glove.

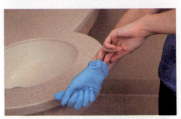

10. Using fingers inserted beneath the glove, roll the glove down over the hand and wrap the other glove within it.

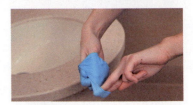

11. Dispose of the gloves and perform hand hygiene.

Source: Pearson Education/PH College.

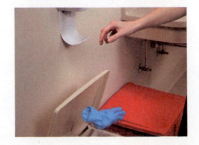

FIGURE 4-9.
Donning and removing sterile gloves.

1. Both gloves are wrapped in a sterile package. Lay the sterile package on a clean surface. Note the label for left and right hands, and orient package with left glove to the left and right glove to the right.

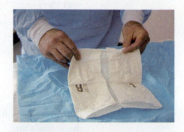

2. Grasp the outer folds of the package and pull apart. Do not touch the inner surface of the package, which is sterile.

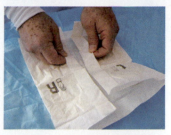

3. Gloves have wrists folded back toward the fingers, which exposes the inner surface of the wrist. Grasp a glove at the base of the wrist area with one hand and insert the fingers of other hand into the glove.

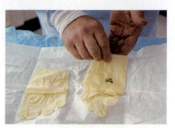

4. Grasping the folded wrist, pull the glove onto the hand. Leave the wrist area folded as it was in the package.

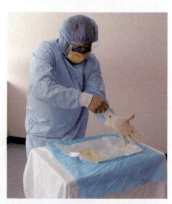

5. Insert gloved fingers inside the folded wrist of the other glove.

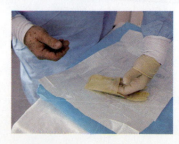

6. Position the glove over the fingertips of the other hand and pull over the hand.

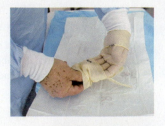

7. Pull the glove on, unfold the wrist, and pull it over the cuff of the gown's arm.

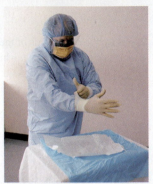

8. Grasp the folded, inverted wrist of the first glove and pull it over the cuff of the gown.

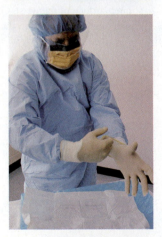

9. The outer surface of the gloves is sterile. Do not touch nonsterile surfaces with these gloves.

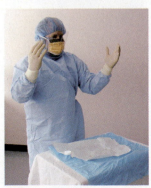

10. To remove, use a gloved hand to grasp the wrist of one glove. Begin to peel it off, turning it inside out.

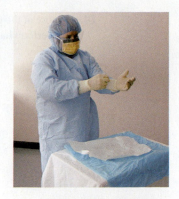

11. Continue to pull glove off and away from the hand.

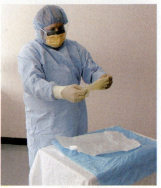

12. Enclose the glove just removed within the palm of the gloved hand.

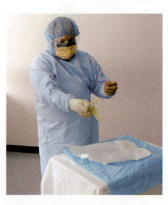

13. Slide the fingers of the bare hand under the wrist of the gloved hand and pull off the glove, enclosing the first glove within it.

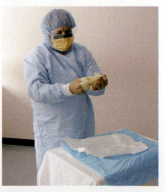

14. Dispose of the gloves, remove other protective equipment, and perform hand hygiene.

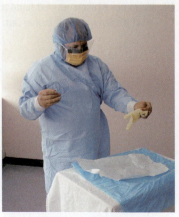

Source: Courtesy of AZIMUTH Incorporated

FIGURE 4-10.

Removing gown and protective gear.

1. To remove gown and protective equipment, begin by untying the straps on the back of the gown.

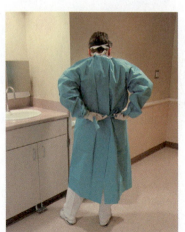

2. Remove gloves and dispose of them.

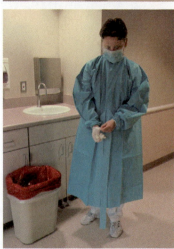

3. Grasp the inner surface of the untied gown at the upper arm or shoulder. Begin to peel off the gown, turning it inside out.

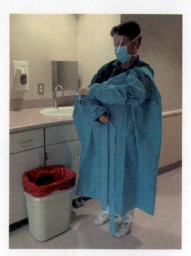

4. Continue to turn the gown inside out and roll it up. Touch only the inside surface of the gown.

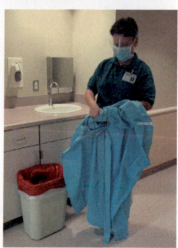

5. Dispose of the gown in a proper biohazard container.

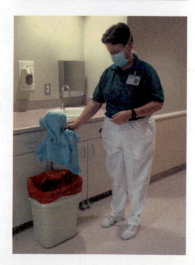

6. Grasp the mask ties behind the head, pull it off, and dispose of it.

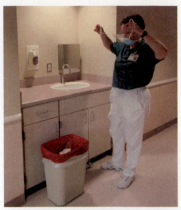

7. Perform hand hygiene with soap and water or alcohol-based hand-rub.

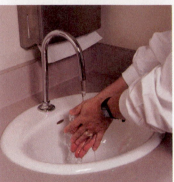

Source: Pearson Education/ PH College

Mouth, Nose, Eye Protection

Certain procedures may produce sprays, splashes, and aerosols that contain blood, body fluids, and other potentially infectious material. Mucous membranes of the eyes, nose, and mouth are vulnerable to infection and require protection during procedures such as bronchoscopy, endotracheal intubation, tracheostomy, catheterization, lumbar puncture, and certain surgical procedures. Note that mouth, nose, and eye PPE is always used for tuberculosis, SARS, and hemorrhagic fever viruses.

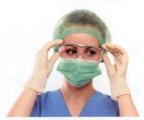

FIGURE 4-11.
Surgical mask. This sterile mask is worn with goggles, gown, and sterile gloves for invasive and surgical procedures.
Source: Sheff/Shutterstock.

Masks are used to protect healthcare workers from infectious respiratory secretions or sprays of body fluids and blood. In general, masks are used if needed as part of transmission-based precautions. Masks are also worn by healthcare workers during procedures that require sterility to protect patients from workers' own potentially infectious material in the mouth and nose. To prevent transmission of infectious respiratory droplets, masks are also placed on coughing patients with respiratory diseases such as measles and tuberculosis. Two types of masks are used in healthcare facilities. The FDA regulates surgical masks, which protect healthcare workers from splashes and respiratory droplets (Figure 4-11). Isolation masks are used for a variety of nonsurgical procedures, but because these are not reviewed by the FDA, they vary in quality and fit. Masks are disposable and

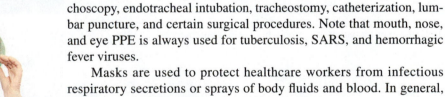

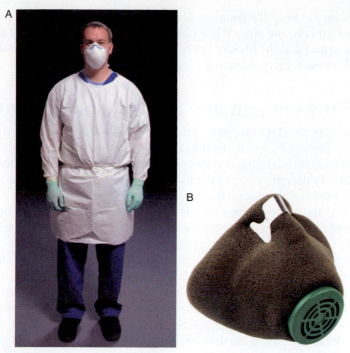

FIGURE 4-12.

Two N95 respirator masks. A respirator similar to these can be used for airborne droplet precautions. Note the fit around the mouth and nose that seals out environmental air.

Source: (A) CDC PHIL and (B) Shutterstock.

are intended for a single use. Masks do not substitute for respirators, which can protect from particulates, the small infectious droplets that are of concern when taking airborne precautions.

Airborne precautions for certain infections such as tuberculosis require the use of respirators for respiratory protection (Figure 4-12). Occupational Safety and Health Administration (OSHA) standards for respiratory protection require that workers get medical approval for wearing a respirator. Employers should provide the correct type of respirator, which currently is an N95 and higher particulate filtering respirator. In addition, employers should give training on correct respirator use and fit-testing on each person required to use a respirator.

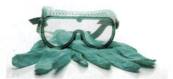

FIGURE 4-13.

Protective eyewear. These goggles will protect the eyes from splashes.

Source: Rob Byron/ Shutterstock.

A variety of goggles and face shields are available for eye protection. Goggles with indirect vents provide the best protection against splashes and particulates (Figure 4-13). These goggles usually fit well over prescription eyeglasses. Safety glasses will not protect from splashes and should not be used for infection control. The mouth, nose, and face are exposed when using goggles, so a mask should be used if it does not interfere with the fit of the goggles. Alternatively, a face shield will comfortably protect the eyes, mouth, and nose. When removing masks, goggles, or face shields, the straps, ties, or material at the back of the head should be grasped because that area of the PPE should remain uncontaminated.

Patient Environment and Medical Instruments

Hand hygiene, PPE, standard precautions, and other well-established practices reduce transmission of pathogens among healthcare workers and patients. In all cases, the practices take into consideration that the patient environment may be contaminated. This section briefly describes steps to reduce the load of pathogens in the patient environment and outlines procedures for disinfecting or sterilizing medical devices and instruments. It is beyond the scope of this text to detail these disinfection and sterilization methods, which may be specified by manufacturer's directions and specific circumstances.

The patient environment is understood to be a clinic waiting room, a clinic examination or procedure room, or a hospital room. Many surfaces are likely to have microorganisms that have been shed by patients and healthcare workers. In an outpatient setting, surfaces with which patients and workers come into contact should be disinfected at regular intervals established by the employer. The surface of the reception desk, the handles on a glass divider or partition at the desk, the telephone, and the waiting room chairs can be contaminated. In outpatient or inpatient treatment areas, surfaces close to the patient or those that the patient has contact with must be cleaned of organic material if necessary and disinfected regularly. Surfaces include bed rails, bed tables, doorknobs, toilet surfaces and toilet room interior. Patient waiting room surfaces should also be disinfected regularly. Pediatric and obstetric-gynecology facilities may have waiting rooms with toys for children. To facilitate regular disinfection, toys with smooth surfaces should be used (i.e., not plush toys or stuffed animals). Disinfectants must have microbiocidal activity against the pathogens expected in the patient environment.

In some cases, medical instruments may be sterile and designed for single use followed by disposal. In other cases, instruments and devices may be reused. These require cleaning and disinfection or sterilization. Good practice requires using a cleaning agent or soap to remove visible soiling and organic material. This facilitates subsequent disinfection and sterilization. Appropriate PPE must be used when disinfecting the environment or medical equipment.

Vaccination

Vaccination protects healthcare workers from many infectious diseases in the workplace. Vaccines stimulate the immune system to recognize and eliminate pathogens and microbial toxins. During an immune response to infection, antibodies and lymphocytes are produced. **Lymphocytes** include B cells and T cells, which reside in lymph nodes, the spleen, and blood. B cells mature during an immune response, turn into plasma cells, and begin producing antibodies. **Antibodies** (also called immunoglobulin) are proteins that recognize specific pathogens or toxins, and by binding to them, help destroy them before they can cause disease. The substance an antibody binds is called an **antigen**, which can be

TABLE 4-5. Healthcare Personnel Vaccination Recommendations

Vaccine	Dosage	Comments
Hepatitis B	3 doses Initial; 2nd dose 1 month after initial; 3rd dose 5 months after 2nd	Obtain anti-HBs serologic testing 1 to 2 months after 3rd dose
Influenza	1 dose annually	Inactivated injectable intradermal or live attenuated influenza vaccine intranasally
Meningococcal meningitis	1 dose annually	For microbiologists who are routinely exposed to cultures of *Neisseria meningitides*
MMR (measles, mumps, rubella)	2 doses, 4 weeks apart	For healthcare personnel born 1957 or later without serologic evidence of immunity or prior vaccination
Tetanus, diphtheria, pertussis	Td booster every 10 years, following the completion of the primary 3-dose series	One dose Tdap for all healthcare personnel younger than 65 years with direct patient contact
Varicella (chickenpox)	2 doses, 4 weeks apart	For healthcare personnel who have no serologic proof of immunity, prior vaccination, or history of varicella disease

Hepatitis A, typhoid, polio: Vaccines are not routinely recommended for healthcare personnel who may have on-the-job exposure to fecal material.

Source: Immunization Action Coalition www.immunize.org

nearly any component of a pathogen. T cells recognize and destroy body cells infected with viruses, which helps control the spread of viruses. A specialized type of T cell is the helper T cell, a cell that controls and coordinates the immune system.

Vaccines usually do not contain living pathogens or active toxins. Instead, vaccines consist of dead microorganisms, inactivated bacterial toxins, bacterial antigens, dead or inactivated viruses, or viral antigens. The vaccine induces an immune response to these substances, which essentially are just parts of pathogens. But the immune system remembers these substances and is capable of responding to subsequent exposures to the whole pathogen. For this reason, several vaccines can protect from infection and are routinely administered to healthcare workers. Vaccines are available for several, but not all, infectious diseases. Table 4-5 ■ lists the names, doses, and recommendations for several vaccines of significance to healthcare workers.

Vaccines have successfully controlled a number of serious infectious diseases, including hepatitis B, measles, tetanus, diphtheria, and pertussis. Vaccination eliminated smallpox from the world and soon will extinguish polio.

WORK SAFE!
Influenza Vaccination Recommendations, 2012

Influenza virus types B and C cause seasonal flu. These viruses change antigens slightly each year, which requires us to annually update vaccine formulations to keep pace with these changes. Thus the updated vaccines protect patients and healthcare workers from virus strains the CDC expects will circulate in the coming season.

Influenza type A viruses pose an entirely different risk. Each year the influenza A viruses can change antigens dramatically (a process named antigenic shift). The human population possesses no immunity to the newly evolved viruses. Thus, influenza A causes epidemics and pandemics. Vaccines protect from these epidemics, but unfortunately the new strains arise rarely and remotely, sometimes escaping surveillance for some time. One such virus was the H1N1 virus identified in May 2009 in Mexico.

CDC recommendations for seasonal influenza vaccination follow below:

- All persons aged 6 months and older should be vaccinated annually.
- Protection of persons at higher risk for influenza-related complications should continue to be a focus of vaccination efforts as providers and programs transition to routine vaccination of all persons aged 6 months and older.
- When vaccine supply is limited, vaccination efforts should focus on delivering vaccination to persons who:
  - are aged 6 months—4 years (59 months);
  - are aged 50 years and older;
  - have chronic pulmonary (including asthma), cardiovascular (except hypertension), renal, hepatic, neurologic, hematologic, or metabolic disorders (including diabetes mellitus);
  - are immunosuppressed (including immunosuppression caused by medications or by human immunodeficiency virus);
  - are or will be pregnant during the influenza season;
  - are aged 6 months—18 years and receiving long-term aspirin therapy and who therefore might be at risk for experiencing Reye syndrome after influenza virus infection;
  - are residents of nursing homes and other chronic-care facilities;
  - are American Indians/Alaska Natives;
  - are morbidly obese (body-mass index is 40 or greater);
  - are healthcare personnel;
  - are household contacts and caregivers of children aged younger than 5 years and adults aged 50 years and older, with particular emphasis on vaccinating contacts of children aged younger than 6 months; and
  - are household contacts and caregivers of persons with medical conditions that put them at higher risk for severe complications from influenza.

Source: Centers for Disease Control and Prevention www.cdc.gov

Chapter Summary

- Infectious diseases and healthcare-associated infections can be controlled.
- Hand hygiene is central to infection control.
- Standard precautions must be practiced with all patients.
- Transmission-based precautions focus on blocking the known transmission methods for each type of infectious disease.
- PPE prevents transmission of infectious diseases.
- Vaccination builds immunity in healthcare workers.

Application

Case Study 4-1: Clean Gloves for Patient Transport?

The employer at your clinic told personnel that it was no longer acceptable for them to wear clean exam gloves while transporting patients, nor was it acceptable to wear clean exam gloves when transporting trash and linen to the decontamination area. The rationale offered for this policy was that if the patients were provided and are using clean gowns and linen, there was no need for gloves. Also, if the trash and linen bags were not soiled, then there was no need for gloves. However, an employee believed that she and her coworkers should protect themselves by using clean gloves during all transport. She was advised by her supervisor that she will be counseled on her behavior should she continue to wear clean exam gloves while performing the previously mentioned duties.

Questions:

1. The employer directive seems at odds with the employee's understanding of the Bloodborne Pathogen standard. Can the employer make this decision? Explain your answer.
2. Should this employee wear new gloves when transporting patients?

Case Study 4-2: Infection Control in the Outpatient Endoscopy Department

The director of your endoscopy office inspected the facility to determine compliance with infection control practices. Her audit revealed opportunities for improving infection control. She directed the following changes in the department:

1. Dispensers for antibacterial hand sanitizers were installed on the wall by the reception desk, next to the building entrances, near every room, and in the hallways.
2. Signs about hand hygiene were posted throughout the facility and in restrooms. The facility's written policy was reviewed and distributed to each employee.
3. Managers audited staff members for hand hygiene compliance.
4. An infection control officer was appointed.
5. Rooms were cleaned at the end of every day. All endoscopy equipment was cleaned and sterilized at the end of each day.
6. Annual safety and infection control training was established.

Questions:

1. Identify which actions are engineering controls, safe work practice, and administrative controls, and which involve PPE.

2. Explain what other infection control measures might be taken in this department.

Assessment

Select the one best answer.

1. Which active ingredient is in most disinfectant hand-rubs?
   a. iodine
   b. bleach
   c. chlorhexidine gluconate
   d. alcohol

2. Which precautions are required for measles and tuberculosis?
   a. standard
   b. contact
   c. airborne
   d. droplet

3. Hand hygiene must be performed:
   a. after removing PPE
   b. after contact with a patient
   c. before preforming a sterile procedure
   d. all of the above
   e. none of the above

4. The fewest number of HAIs occur in which of these settings?
   a. home care
   b. long-term care
   c. hospital
   d. ambulatory care

5. Which statement about vaccines is correct?
   a. Vaccines are available for most infections.
   b. Vaccines are composed of living microorganisms.
   c. Vaccines work by making someone sick to stimulate immunity.
   d. Vaccines are a highly effective and a safe way to stimulate protective immunity.

Resources

American Society for Microbiology www.asm.org
Centers for Disease Control and Prevention www.cdc.gov
Advisory Committee and the HICPAC/SHEA/APIC/IDSA Hand Hygiene Task Force. *Guideline for Hand Hygiene in Health-Care Settings Recommendations of the Healthcare Infection Control Practices.* Centers for Disease Control and Prevention, MMWR, 2002. Recommendations and Reports Vol. 51.

Siegel JD, Rhinehart E, Jackson M, Chiarello L, and the Healthcare Infection Control Practices Advisory Committee, Centers for Disease Control and Prevention. 2007. *Guideline for Isolation Precautions: Preventing Transmission of Infectious Agents in Healthcare Settings.* Centers for Disease Control and Prevention.

WHO Guidelines on Hand Hygiene in Healthcare, 2009. World Health Organization. World Health Organization www.who.org

CHAPTER 5

Blood-Borne Pathogens

This chapter describes the Bloodborne Pathogens Standard, explains the risks associated with blood-borne pathogens, and describes best practices for preventing their transmission.

Objectives

After completing this chapter, the student will be able to:

- Understand and apply the Bloodborne Pathogens Standard.
- Describe how blood-borne pathogens are transmitted.
- Understand the components of standard precautions.
- Understand the components of an exposure control plan.
- Know the engineering, work practice, and personal protective equipment (PPE) controls for blood-borne pathogens.
- Know best practice for safe handling and disposal of needles and biohazardous waste.
- Understand the importance of follow-up and prophylaxis after exposure to blood-borne pathogens.

Key Terms and Concepts

antiretroviral medication
blood-borne pathogen
cirrhosis
exposure control plan
hepatitis B vaccine
hepatitis B virus (HBV)

hepatitis C virus (HCV)
human immunodeficiency
  virus (HIV)
postexposure prophylaxis
safe injection practice
standard precautions

The Bloodborne Pathogens Standard

The Occupational Safety and Health Administration (OSHA) Bloodborne Pathogens Standard is designed to protect healthcare workers from exposure to pathogenic microorganisms that are present in human blood and other body fluids. The pathogens of concern include human immunodeficiency virus (HIV), hepatitis B, and hepatitis C, all of which can be transmitted in blood and other body fluids. In the years after the standard was implemented and the hepatitis B vaccine was introduced, the incidence of workplace-acquired **blood-borne pathogen** infection dropped dramatically. The incidence of these infections remains low wherever blood-borne pathogen controls are practiced.

Human Immunodeficiency Virus and Hepatitis Viruses

Blood and other body fluids may transmit several types of pathogens, but the chief pathogens of concern are human immunodeficiency virus (HIV), hepatitis B virus (HBV), and hepatitis C virus (HCV) because these viruses can cause chronic, life-threatening disease. Fortunately, measures that control exposure to these three viruses also block transmission of other blood-borne pathogens.

Human Immunodeficiency Virus

Human immunodeficiency virus (HIV) infects T cells and other cells of the body, cripples the immune system, and renders the host susceptible to opportunistic infectious diseases and tumors. HIV-related diseases include tuberculosis, *Pneumocystis* pneumonia, and Kaposi's sarcoma. No effective HIV vaccine exists, but **antiretroviral medications** target HIV's ability to replicate and reproduce in human cells. By controlling HIV's growth, it is possible to live with HIV as a chronic infection.

HIV is transmitted in blood, semen, vaginal fluids, breast milk, as well as by hypodermic needles, transfusions, and sexual contact. In the healthcare setting, all other body fluids are considered potentially infectious. Since 1991, the Centers for Disease Control and Prevention (CDC) has formally investigated cases of HIV infection in healthcare workers and requires state and local health departments to do so as well. As a result, many data are available that describe the risks of becoming infected in the workplace. Although HIV is a notifiable infectious disease for health departments and healthcare workers, individuals are not required to report their occupational exposure, and thus it is likely that cases remain underreported. Occupational exposure to HIV is documented when an exposed healthcare worker shows seroconversion (the development of antibodies) following an exposure event and has no other nonoccupational risk factors for HIV exposure.

In the United States between 1981 and 2006, fifty-seven healthcare workers showed seroconversion (developed antibodies to HIV) and did not have nonoccupational risk factors. Exposure occurred through a few routes. Most of these workers, 48 of 57, sustained percutaneous injuries such as needle sticks or cuts. Five were exposed through mucous membranes, two were exposed through both percutaneous injury and mucous membranes, and two were exposed through an unknown route. Blood exposure occurred in 49 cases, exposure to other body fluids occurred in five cases, and exposure to concentrated virus in the laboratory occurred in three cases. According to the CDC, the last probable healthcare-related exposure occurred in 2009. A few other exposures are currently under investigation. The CDC reports that the risk for acquiring HIV occupationally is extremely low and that most exposures do not result in HIV infection. In addition, a study of worldwide needle-stick–related HIV found an average transmission rate of 0.3% per needle-stick injury. More than 90% of healthcare workers do have nonoccupational exposure to HIV (multiple sex partners, intravenous drug use, for example), however, which makes it difficult to pinpoint the workplace as the site of exposure.

Hepatitis B Virus

The **hepatitis B virus (HBV)** infects the liver, causing a variety of systemic symptoms that include fever, fatigue, loss of appetite, nausea, vomiting, abdominal pain, joint pain, and jaundice. More serious is the risk for chronic infection, which may lead to **cirrhosis**, liver cancer, liver failure, and death. Each year in the United States, about 43,000 new HBV infections and 3,000 HBV-related deaths occur; consequently, it is important for healthcare workers to take precautions. HBV is transmitted by blood from an infected person. This can occur during any procedure involving blood exposure but is usually associated with needle sticks, cuts, and transfusions. Fortunately, the **hepatitis B vaccine** is extremely effective (more on vaccines later in this chapter). For example, one study found that vaccinated healthcare workers are well protected from needle-stick injury–associated HBV, and their risk of becoming infected with the virus is virtually nonexistent.

Hepatitis C Virus

The **hepatitis C virus (HCV)** also infects the liver. In contrast to HBV, 85% of HCV infections are chronic, with most of these chronic infections leading to chronic liver disease, cirrhosis, or liver cancer. Up to 5% of people infected with HCV die from liver cancer or cirrhosis; each year, 12,000 persons die from HCV-related illness. With 17,000 new infections each year in the United States and no available vaccine, this disease should be of concern to healthcare workers. However, the risk for occupation-related infection is relatively low. For example, the risk following exposure to infected blood via needle stick is about 1.8%. The incidence of occupation-related HCV remains unknown. The incidence of HCV infection in the community is 1.6%; the incidence is 1% among healthcare workers. Other than needle-stick data, no information is available to accurately describe the overall incidence of occupation-related HCV.

Exposure Control Plan

The Bloodborne Pathogens Standard requires employers to develop, distribute, and implement an **exposure control plan**. The exposure control plan identifies employees who may be exposed to blood-borne pathogens by virtue of their work. The plan then describes engineering controls, work practice, personal protective equipment (PPE), employee training, hazard communication, postexposure measures, and recordkeeping requirements.

Engineering Controls

Engineering controls include physical methods that prevent blood-borne pathogens from entering the workplace or that isolate hazards from workers. The most significant of these are disposal containers for needles and other sharps (see Figure 1-3), self-sheathing needles, and devices such as needleless injection systems. Needle safety is discussed later in this chapter. Biosafety cabinets for contained laboratory work with pathogens may be used as well (see Figure 1-4).

WORDS OF WARNING!
Sharps Container Hazards

The majority of needle-stick injuries occur after use and during disposal. Needles inside a sharps container that is more than three-quarters full can interfere with the opening and block the addition of more needles. Take these precautions:

1. Before beginning a procedure, ensure the room has a sharps container with capacity for more needles.
2. Do not use a full sharps container.
3. Do not carry a needle to another room for disposal.
4. Do not force a needle into a sharps container.
5. If sharps containers are not affixed to the wall, they should be placed on counters within comfortable reach so that you make no awkward movements during disposal.
6. Remember: Never recap needles.

Standard Precautions

Recall that needle sticks and direct contact with blood are associated with the vast majority of occupationally acquired HIV infections. It follows, then, that the most important work practices for controlling blood-borne pathogens are **standard precautions** and needle safety.

Standard precautions were published in the CDC's *Guidelines for Isolation Precautions in Hospitals* (1983) to replace the organization's former *Blood and Body Fluid Precautions* and in response to the emerging occupational hazards of blood-borne pathogens, specifically HIV, HBV, and HCV.

Chapter 4 discusses standard precautions, first described by the CDC in 1996. Standard precautions apply mainly in hospital settings and are designed to protect patients and workers from a wide range of infectious diseases. In contrast, universal precautions apply in all healthcare, first aid, and emergency situations, inside or outside of healthcare facilities. The premise of universal precautions is that *blood and other body fluids of all patients should be considered potentially infectious for HIV, HBV, and HCV.*

Blood-borne pathogens are not found only in blood. However, they do not occur in all other body fluids and secretions. Standard precautions should be observed when the following are in the healthcare setting: semen, vaginal secretions, and blood and other body fluids that contain visible blood. Standard precautions also apply to tissues and body cavity fluids such as cerebrospinal, synovial, pleural, peritoneal, pericardial, and amniotic fluids. Blood-borne pathogens are not found in feces, nasal secretions, sputum, sweat, tears, urine, or vomitus unless they contain visible blood; if these materials contain visible blood, standard precautions apply. Likewise, standard precautions do not apply to saliva except when it is visibly contaminated with blood or in the dental setting where blood contamination of saliva is normally expected. Table 5-1 ■ describes the components of standard precautions.

TABLE 5-1. Standard Precautions

Component	Indications
Gloves, general	Touching blood and other body fluids, mucous membranes, or nonintact skin of all patients. Handling items or surfaces soiled with blood or other body fluids.
Gloves, phlebotomy	Performing phlebotomy when the healthcare worker has cuts, scratches, or other breaks in his or her skin. In situations where the healthcare worker judges that hand contamination with blood may occur, for example, when performing phlebotomy on an uncooperative patient. Performing finger- and/or heel-sticks on infants and children. When persons are receiving training in phlebotomy.
Gowns or aprons	During procedures that are likely to generate droplets or splashes of blood or other body fluids.
Masks and protective eyeware	During procedures likely to generate droplets or splashes of blood or other body fluids to prevent exposure of mucous membranes of the mouth, nose, and eyes.
Safe needle and other sharps practice	During procedures. When cleaning used instruments. During disposal of used needles. When handling sharp instruments after procedures. To prevent needle-stick injuries, *needles should never be recapped by hand*, purposely bent or broken by hand, removed from disposable syringes, or otherwise manipulated by hand. After they are used, disposable syringes and needles, scalpel blades, and other sharp items should be placed in puncture-resistant containers for disposal. The puncture-resistant containers should be located as close as practical to the use area. All reusable needles should be placed in a puncture-resistant container for transport to the reprocessing area.

Sources: Centers for Disease Control and Prevention (CDC). Guidelines for prevention of transmission of human immunodeficiency virus and hepatitis B virus to health-care and public-safety workers. *MMWR* 1989;38(S-6):1–36.

Centers for Disease Control and Prevention (CDC). Recommendations for prevention of HIV transmission in health-care settings. *MMWR* 1987;36(S-2S)pp. 1–18.

Centers for Disease Control and Prevention (CDC). Update: Universal precautions for prevention of transmission of human immunodeficiency virus, hepatitis B virus, and other bloodborne pathogens in health-care settings. *MMWR* 1988;37:377–388.

Injection, Needle, and Other Sharps Safety

According to the CDC, more than 8 million healthcare workers in the United States sustain 600,000 to 800,000 needle-stick injuries each year. One might expect such a large number of injuries to result in a large number of blood-borne pathogen–related infections, but as discussed earlier, that is not the case.

Though needle-stick–associated HIV is extremely rare, 85% of occupationally acquired HIV infections are caused by needle-stick injuries. Hence, preventing needle-stick injuries and observing sharps safety can significantly reduce the incidence of occupation-related HIV infections. A good resource for needle-stick safety is the National Institute for Occupational Safety and Health (NIOSH). NIOSH is a branch of the CDC and is responsible for preventing workplace injuries and accidents.

Safe practices should extend at all times to all sharp devices, including hypodermic needles, blood collection needles, intravenous (IV) stylets, and needles used to connect parts of IV delivery systems. Each of these devices can cause percutaneous injuries, 80% of which occur during and after use but before disposal. The majority of needle-stick injuries occur during disposal into sharps containers that are full or when reaching into a full sharps container to deposit a needle. In these cases, workers' hands become injured by contaminated needles at the mouth of the full container. It is important to replace sharps containers before they become filled to the top and to ensure that empty containers are available before beginning a procedure. Many injuries also occur when taking apart and otherwise handling needle assemblies or phlebotomy needle and vacuum tube devices. Needlestick injuries can also occur during the cumbersome disposal of needles attached to flexible tubing. Additional causes of needle-stick injuries include recapping needles, transferring body fluid between containers, and failure to dispose used needles in puncture-resistant sharps containers. An important way to reduce needle-stick injuries is to develop and use safer needle devices such as those that retract needles into protective sheaths (Figures 5-1, 5-2, 5-3, and 5-4). Table 5-2 ■ describes other needle safety practices.

Related to safe needle practice is **safe injection practice**. Safe injection practice applies to vaccination; spinal procedures, including myelogram, lumbar puncture, spinal and epidural anesthesia, and intrathecal chemotherapy; administration of parenteral medication; and blood draws. The CDC describes safe injection practices that apply to the use of needles, cannulas that replace needles, and IV delivery systems (Table 5-3 ■).

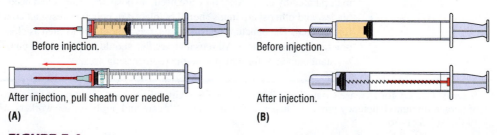

Before injection.   Before injection.

After injection, pull sheath over needle.   After injection.

(A)   **(B)**

FIGURE 5-1.

Needle safety. Syringes with safety features. *Source*: Giangrasso, Dosage Calculations, Figure 7.35 (Pearson).

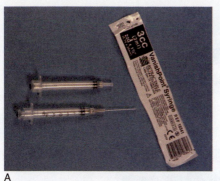
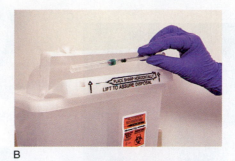
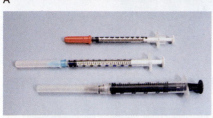
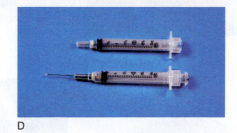

A

B

C

D

FIGURE 5-2.
Needle-stick safety. (A) Safety needles. (B) Syringes are discarded in a biohazard container. (C) Tuberculin, insulin, and 3-mL syringes. (D) Safety syringe with a retractable needle and a needle retracted into the barrel. *Source*: Pearson Education/PH College.

A

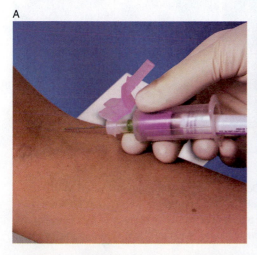
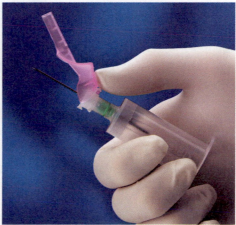

(A) BD Eclipse blood collection needle attached to a holder (courtesy and copyright Becton, Dickinson and Company)
FIGURE 5-3.
Safety syringes.

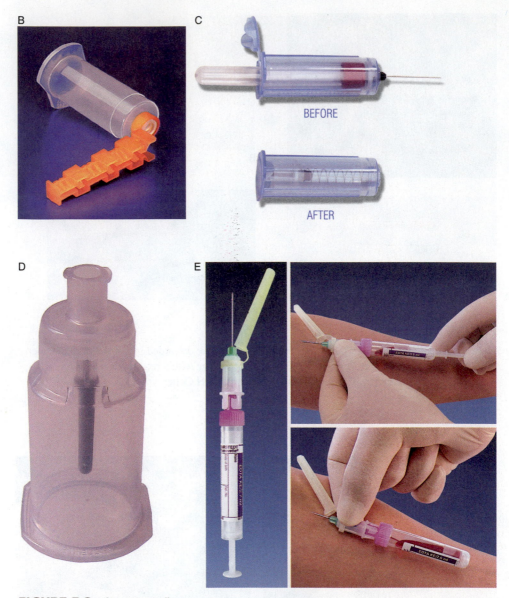

FIGURE 5-3. *(Continued)*

(B) Venipuncture needle-Pro Needle Protection Device (courtesy of Smiths Medical/ASD, Inc, Carlsbad, CA. (C) Vanishpoint blood collection tube holder (courtesy of Retractable Technologies, Little Elm, TX). (D) Vacuette Quickshield safety tube holder (courtesy of Grenier Bio-One, GmbH, Kremsmuenster, Austria). (E) Sarstedt S-Monovette venous blood collection system (courtesy of Sarstedt, Inc., Newton, NC).

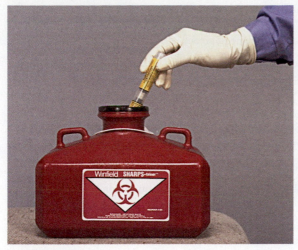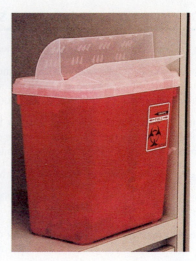

FIGURE 5-4.
Sharps containers.
Source: Pearson Education/PH College.

TABLE 5-2. National Institute of Occupational Safety and Health (NIOSH)
Recommendations for Preventing Needle-Stick Injuries

Avoid the use of needles where safe and effective alternatives are available.

Help your employer select and evaluate devices with safety features.

Use devices with safety features provided by your employer.

Never recap needles.

Plan for safe handling and disposal before beginning any procedure using needles.

Dispose of used needles promptly in appropriate sharps disposal containers.

Report all needle-stick and other sharps-related injuries promptly to ensure that you receive appropriate follow-up care.

Tell your employer about needle hazards that you observe in your work environment.

Participate in blood-borne pathogen training and follow recommended infection prevention practices, including hepatitis B vaccination.

Source: National Institute for Occupational Safety and Health (NIOSH) Alert: *Preventing Needlestick Injuries in Healthcare Settings*. DHHS (NIOSH) Publication No. 2000.108.NIOSH. 1999

Documented lapses in safe injection practice have caused numerous infections. Recent transmissions of blood-borne pathogens were traced to the use of medication vials for multiple patients and the reuse of syringes (following needle disposal). Also, cases of bacterial meningitis have occurred following procedures involving lumbar puncture. Healthcare workers should wear masks during such procedures to prevent transmission of oropharyngeal pathogens (e.g., the bacteria that cause meningitis). This recommendation appears in the current CDC injection safety recommendations and is among the revised standard precautions (see Chapter 4).

TABLE 5-3. CDC Recommendations for Safe Injection Practices

Use aseptic technique to avoid contamination of sterile injection equipment.

Do not administer medications from a syringe to multiple patients, even if the needle or cannula on the syringe is changed. Needles, cannulae and syringes are sterile, single-use items; they should not be reused for another patient nor to access a medication or solution that might be used for a subsequent patient.

Use fluid infusion and administration sets (e.g., IV bags, tubing, and connectors) for one patient only and dispose appropriately after use. Consider a syringe or needle/cannula contaminated once it has been used to enter or connect to a patient's IV infusion bag or administration set.

Use single-dose vials for parenteral medications whenever possible.

Do not administer medications from single-dose vials or ampules to multiple patients or combine leftover contents for later use.

If multidose vials must be used, both the needle or cannula and syringe used to access the multidose vial must be sterile.

Do not keep multidose vials in the immediate patient treatment area. Store them in accordance with the manufacturer's recommendations. Discard if sterility is compromised or questionable.

Do not use bags or bottles of IV solution as a common source of supply for multiple patients.

Source: Centers for Disease Control and Prevention (CDC). *2007 Guideline for Isolation Precautions: Preventing Transmission of Infectious Agents in Healthcare Settings.* 2007 Centers for Disease Control and Prevention

Personal Protective Equipment for Blood-Borne Pathogens

An employer's blood-borne pathogen exposure control plan should also prescribe the use of appropriate personal protective equipment (PPE) under circumstances in which exposure is likely. Employers must make gloves, masks, face shields, eyewear, and gowns easily available; maintain them in good repair; and train employees on correct use. PPE is discussed in detail in Chapter 4.

Vaccination

Employers must offer the HBV vaccine to healthcare employees within 10 days of hiring, unless the employee has evidence of prior vaccination. Healthcare employees can decline the vaccine. Employees must sign a waiver stating that the vaccine was offered, they declined, and they understand the risks of exposure to HBV.

The HBV vaccine contains hepatitis B virus surface antigen (HBsAg), and protective immunity is indicated when a person develops anti-HBs antibodies. Healthcare workers whose work may expose them to blood or other body fluids should receive three doses of HBV vaccine at 0-, 1-, and 6-month intervals. One to two months after the third dose, immunity should be confirmed by measuring anti-HBs antibodies. If immunity is not detected, the three-dose vaccination should be repeated. If no immunity is detected after this sixth vaccine dose, the person is described as a nonresponder and should be considered unprotected against HBV. Nonresponders need to take all normal precautions to prevent HBV infection. They must be advised to obtain immunoglobulin prophylaxis following known or possible exposure to HBV.

> ## WORK SAFE!
> ## HBV Vaccine
>
> The HBV vaccine has proven to be extremely effective. Those who have received the hepatitis B vaccine and demonstrate immunity to the virus have virtually no risk for infection. In contrast, an unvaccinated person's risk from a needle-stick exposure to HBV-infected blood is 6 to 30%. It is hard to understate the impact of this vaccine. Annual occupational infections have decreased 95% since the hepatitis B vaccine became available in 1982.

No vaccines exist for HIV and HCV. Therefore, HIV and HCV infection control relies on observing standard precautions and on **postexposure prophylaxis**.

Postexposure Follow-Up and Prophylaxis

Should an employee be exposed to blood-borne pathogens, the employer must provide—at no cost to the worker—postexposure follow-up and prophylaxis. Employees can waive their right to follow-up and prophylaxis. Laboratory tests should be conducted to determine if exposure resulted in infection, and prophylactic medication should be provided following exposure. HIV, HBV, or HCV exposures each require different follow-up and prophylaxis (Table 5-4 ■). Employers must provide exposed employees with counseling because often, considerable stress is associated with exposure. Employers should consult the Post-Exposure Prophylaxis Hotline (PEPline) at 888-448-4911. This is a support system that provides guidelines and other resources for clinicians who treat and counsel employees who have been exposed to blood-borne pathogens.

Hazard Communication and Hazardous Waste

Signs and labels bearing the standard biohazard symbol must be used to clearly identify hazards in the workplace (Figure 5-5). Signs should identify restricted areas as well as refrigerators and freezers where hazardous waste and potentially infectious material are stored. Labels should be affixed to all containers used to store blood, blood products, discarded sharps, and any infectious material.

There is no evidence that current medical waste storage and disposal practices have caused disease among healthcare employees (except of course the infections caused by contaminated needles, which usually occur before disposal and storage). Different types of waste pose different degrees of threat to health; therefore, it is impractical to treat all medical waste as if it were dangerous. As a result, federal, state, and local regulations have classified medical waste to identify the types of waste that require precautions during storage, handling, and transport. Such waste is called regulated waste and includes blood and body fluid

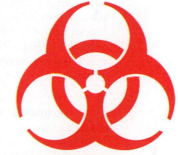

FIGURE 5-5.

Universal biohazard symbol. This symbol indicates the possible presence of blood, blood products, or other material hazardous to human health. This symbol should be visible on sharps containers, storage containers, and biohazard bags, and in work areas where such hazards exist.

Source: CDC.

TABLE 5-4. Postexposure Response for Blood-Borne Pathogens

Components of Postexposure Response	HIV	HBV	HCV
Postexposure Vaccine	No. None available.	Yes. HBV immune globulin plus HBV vaccine if unvaccinated.	No. None available.
Prophylactic Drugs	Yes. Four-week course of a two-drug antiretroviral cocktail or three-drug antiretroviral cocktail if higher risk (exposure to large amount of virus or drug-resistant virus).	Yes. HBV immune globulin plus HBV vaccine if unvaccinated or if a nonresponder.	No effective drugs available.
Timing	As soon as possible following exposure.	As soon as possible following exposure. Less than 24 hours and not more than 7 days.	No effective drugs available.
Drug Safety and Adverse Effects	Adverse effects are common and include nausea, vomiting, diarrhea, tiredness, headache. Some may suffer from kidney stones, hepatitis, anemia, leucopenia. Protease inhibitors interact with other medicines (e.g., nonsedating antihistamines) and may cause serious adverse effects.	Vaccine and immune globulin are safe and tolerated well.	No effective drugs available.
Follow-Up	Test for HIV antibody as soon as possible following exposure. Before and during antiretroviral therapy, get complete blood count (CBC), test kidney and liver function. Monitor for signs and symptoms of HIV infection.	None recommended.	Test for HCV antibody and measure liver enzyme level (ALT) four to six weeks following exposure.
Precautions During Follow-Up	Six to twelve weeks postexposure, refrain from donating blood, practice safe sex, always use a condom, mothers should avoid breastfeeding.	None recommended because vaccination is highly effective.	None recommended because risk of acquiring and transmitting HCV is very low.

Source: Centers for Disease Control and Prevention (CDC). *Exposure to Blood: What Healthcare Personnel Need to Know.* 2003 www.cdc.gov

specimens, needles, other sharps, microbiology laboratory waste, pathology laboratory waste, and human anatomy waste (e.g., surgery and autopsy waste).

To minimize transport and exposure, such medical waste should be disposed of near the point it is generated. Medical waste must be contained in sturdy, leak-resistant, sealable red biohazard bags that can be stored in bright red or orange leak-proof, puncture-proof containers until it leaves the facility. State and local regulations regarding waste treatment and disinfection vary. In some communities, waste is autoclaved or incinerated on-site before it leaves the facility.

Training

Employers must identify all employees whose work exposes them to blood-borne pathogens and provide training upon hire and annually. Training topics must include the hazards of blood-borne pathogens, preventive practices, and postexposure procedures.

Records and Reporting

Follow-up must include incident reporting. OSHA requires that employers maintain a five-year log of workplace injuries and illnesses. The log should record the date of the incident, the department in which the incident occurred, an explanation of how the exposure occurred, and a description of any medical devices related to the exposure. Incidents related to sharps injuries should be recorded on OSHA form 300 (Box 5-1 ■).

Employers must also maintain employee medical records, training records, and sharps injury logs. Employees must report all needle-stick and other sharps injuries as well as other occupational injuries. In addition, employees must be given access to their records upon request.

BOX 5-1. OSHA Form 300. Workplace sharps injuries must be reported on this log.

OSHA's Form 300 (Rev. 01/2004)

Log of Work-Related Injuries and Illnesses

Attention: This form contains information relating to employee health and must be used in a manner that protects the confidentiality of employees to the extent possible while the information is being used for occupational safety and health purposes.

Year 20____

U.S. Department of Labor
Occupational Safety and Health Administration

Form approved OMB no. 1218-0176

You must record information about every work-related death and about every work-related injury or illness that involves loss of consciousness, restricted work activity or job transfer, days away from work, or medical treatment beyond first aid. You must also record significant work-related injuries and illnesses that are diagnosed by a physician or licensed health care professional. You must also record work-related injuries and illnesses that meet any of the specific recording criteria listed in 29 CFR Part 1904.8 through 1904.12. Feel free to use two lines for a single case if you need to. You must complete an injury and illness Incident Report (OSHA Form 301) or equivalent form for each injury or illness recorded on this form. If you're not sure whether a case is recordable, call your local OSHA office for help.

Establishment name _____

City _____ State _____

Identify the person

(A) Case no.	(B) Employee's name	(C) Job title (e.g., Welder)

Describe the case

(D) Date of injury or onset of illness	(E) Where the event occurred (e.g., Loading dock north end)	(F) Describe injury or illness, parts of body affected, and object/substance that directly injured or made person ill (e.g., Second degree burns on right forearm from acetylene torch)

Classify the case

CHECK ONLY ONE box for each case based on the most serious outcome for that case:

| | Remained at Work | | |
| Death (G) | Days away from work (H) | Job transfer or restriction (I) | Other recordable cases (J) |

Enter the number of days the injured or ill worker was:

| Away from work (K) days | On job transfer or restriction (L) days |

Check the "Injury" column or choose one type of illness:
(M)

| Injury (1) | Skin disorder (2) | Respiratory condition (3) | Poisoning (4) | Hearing loss (5) | All other Illnesses (6) |

Page totals ▶

Be sure to transfer these totals to the Summary page (Form 300A) before you post it.

Public reporting burden for this collection of information is estimated to average 14 minutes per response, including time to review the instructions, search and gather the data needed, and complete and review the collection of information. Persons are not required to respond to the collection of information unless it displays a currently valid OMB control number. If you have any comments about these estimates or any other aspects of this data collection, contact: US Department of Labor, OSHA Office of Statistical Analysis, Room N-3644, 200 Constitution Avenue, NW, Washington, DC 20210. Do not send the completed forms to this office.

Page ____ of ____

Chapter Summary

- OSHA's Bloodborne Pathogens Standard protects healthcare workers.
- Human immunodeficiency virus (HIV) and hepatitis viruses can be transmitted by blood and other body fluids.
- An employer's blood-borne pathogen exposure control plan describes how employees will be protected from transmission of pathogens.
- Standard precautions must be practiced with all patients.
- Safe needle practice and safe injection practice help prevent injuries and transmission of pathogens.
- The hepatitis virus B (HBV) vaccination is highly effective.
- Personal protective equipment (PPE) reduces the risk of infection when exposure to blood and other body fluids is likely.
- If exposed to blood-borne pathogens, workers must have postexposure prophylaxis and follow-up.
- Infectious waste must be handled in accordance with OSHA and employer regulations.

Application

Case Study 5-1: Needle-Stick Exposure to HIV

A medical office assistant was preparing an examination room for the next patient. When she picked up paper towels on the floor to dispose in the trash, she punctured her thumb with a needle that was loosely wrapped in the towels. Because this clinic is an outpatient HIV/AIDS clinic, she was very worried about being exposed to HIV.

Questions:

1. Describe how this exposure could have been prevented.
2. How do we know if she acquired HIV?

Case Study 5-2: Selecting PPE for Blood-Borne Pathogens

At the orthopedic clinic where you work, you prepare patients for their examinations. Your next patient is scheduled for a follow-up exam for her hand surgery. After asking the patient a few routine questions, you take her weight and blood pressure. You then change her surgical wound dressing.

Questions:

1. Apply your knowledge of transmission-based precautions and blood-borne pathogens to explain which PPE you need to use during this scenario.
2. Which PPE is not needed?

Assessment

Select the one best answer.

1. The Bloodborne Pathogens Standard covers all of these pathogens except _____ .
   a. human immunodeficiency virus
   b. methicillin-resistant *Staphylococcus aureus*
   c. hepatitis C virus
   d. hepatitis B virus
   e. all of the above are normally transmitted in blood

2. A vaccine is available for _____ .
   a. human immunodeficiency virus
   b. methicillin-resistant *S. aureus*
   c. hepatitis C virus
   d. hepatitis B virus
   e. none of the above

3. When cleaning or inserting a patient's central catheter line, you should wear _____ .
   a. gloves
   b. mask
   c. eye protection
   d. gown
   e. all of the above

4. You should wear gloves when performing which of these procedures?
   a. measuring oral temperature
   b. measuring pulse
   c. administering an influenza vaccine
   d. performing all procedures
   e. none of the above

5. For healthcare workers, most occupational exposure to HIV occurs following _____ .
   a. needle-stick injuries
   b. blood contact with skin
   c. blood or body fluid contact with eyes
   d. blood or body fluid contact with respiratory membranes
   e. none of the above

Resources

American National Standards Institute www.ansi.org
Association for Professionals in Infection Control and Epidemiology www.apic.org
Centers for Disease Control and Prevention (CDC). *Guideline for Isolation Precautions: Preventing Transmission of Infectious Agents in Healthcare Settings*. 2007 Centers for Disease Control and Prevention.
Centers for Disease Control and Prevention (CDC). *Exposure to Blood: What Healthcare Personnel Need to Know*. Centers for Disease Control and Prevention 2003
Centers for Disease Control and Prevention (CDC). Guidelines for prevention of

transmission of human immunodeficiency virus and hepatitis B virus to health-care and public-safety workers. *MMWR* 1989;38(S-6):1-36.

Centers for Disease Control and Prevention (CDC). Recommendations for prevention of HIV transmission in health-care settings. *MMWR* 1987;36(S-2Spp 3-37).

Centers for Disease Control and Prevention (CDC). Update: Universal precautions for prevention of transmission of human immunodeficiency virus, hepatitis B virus, and other bloodborne pathogens in health-care settings. *MMWR* 1988;37:377–388.

National Institute for Occupational Safety and Health www.niosh.gov

National Institute for Occupational Safety and Health (NIOSH) Alert: *Preventing Needle-stick Injuries in Healthcare Settings*. DHHS (NIOSH) Publication No. 2000.108.

Occupational Safety and Health Administration www.osha.gov

PEARSON
myhealthprofessionskit

Visit www.myhealthprofessionskit.com to access the interactive Companion Website for this textbook. Simply select "Basic Health Science" from the choice of disciplines. Find this book and log in using your user name and password to access additional learning tools.

CHAPTER 6

Chemical Safety: Best Practices

This chapter describes the best practices for safely handling, dispensing, storing, and disposing of chemicals commonly found in the healthcare workplace. Personal protective equipment and standard operating procedures are described.

Objectives

After completing this chapter, the student will be able to:

- Describe the Occupational Safety and Health Administration (OSHA) chemical safety standards that apply to the healthcare workplace.
- List the elements of a chemical hygiene and safety plan.
- Explain the hazards associated with chemicals commonly found in the healthcare workplace.
- Describe best practices for safely handling, storing, dispensing, and disposing of chemicals commonly found in the healthcare workplace.

Key Terms and Concepts

anticancer agents
chemical hygiene officer
chemical hygiene plan
ethylene oxide
Ethylene Oxide standard
formaldehyde
Formaldehyde standard
formalin
glutaraldehyde
Hazard Communication standard

hazardous drugs
latex
latex gloves
Material Safety Data Sheet (MSDS)
mercury
nitrile gloves
Occupational Exposure to Hazardous Chemicals in the Laboratory standard

OSHA Standards for Hazardous Chemicals

Healthcare workers must take precautions to prevent exposure to hazardous chemicals in their workplace. Occupational Safety and Health Administration (OSHA) standards require employers to communicate these hazards; describe how to safely handle, store, dispense, and dispose of hazardous chemicals; train employees in best safety practices; and monitor the workplace and employees for exposures. The OSHA **Occupational Exposure to Hazardous Chemicals in the Laboratory standard** applies to the workplace if chemicals are used in laboratory settings. The **Hazard Communication standard** focuses on all aspects of chemical hazard communication and prevention.

The Occupational Exposure to Hazardous Chemicals in the Laboratory standard requires employers to write and implement a **chemical hygiene plan**. The National Research Council describes elements of a practical and effective chemical hygiene plan (Table 6-1 ■) that meets the OSHA standard. Employees probably will not need to access the chemical hygiene plan daily for routine work, but they should be able to obtain the **Material Safety Data Sheet (MSDS)** for each chemical in the workplace. The employer must file and make available the MSDS for each chemical. The MSDS describes a chemical's physical and chemical properties—including flammability and toxicity—and describes safe storage, handling, and personal protective equipment (PPE) (Figure 6-1).

The chemical hygiene plan must describe standard operating procedures for safe handling of hazardous chemicals. For example, if a facility uses glutaraldehyde for disinfection or x-ray development, the plan will spell out standard procedures for how to safely handle, dispense, store, and dispose it.

The plan also describes how the employer will determine the need for the use of certain safety measures such as engineering controls and PPE. Specifically, the employer will describe how to use fume hoods, goggles, gloves, or respirators. If these protections are warranted, the employer will require and provide training on their use.

In addition, the plan must provide for comprehensive employee training and describe the information employees must have about hazardous chemicals. The plan will describe circumstances in which a hazardous procedure (perhaps one that poses special risks) will

TABLE 6-1. Elements of a Chemical Hygiene Plan

Procedures for storage, handling, dispensing, and disposal of hazardous chemicals

Use of personal protective equipment

Use of engineering controls such as fume hoods

Procedures for employee safety training

Procedures for inspection and maintenance of safety equipment

Procedures for record keeping

Provisions for medical consultation in the event of exposure

Methods for hazard communication such as signs, labels, and MSDS

Methods for containing spills and exposures

Assignment of a Chemical Hygiene Officer

Source: Occupational Safety and Health Administration (OSHA). http://www.osha.gov/OshDoc/data_General_Facts/hazardouschemicalsinlabs-factsheet.html

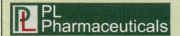

MATERIAL SAFETY DATA SHEET (MSDS)

PL Pharmaceuticals
123 Main Street
Saddle River, NJ 07458
201-555-5555

SECTION 1- CHEMICAL PRODUCT INFORMATION

Sodium Hypochlorite Solution (Bleach)
Manufacturer Name PL Pharmaceuticals

SECTION 2 – COMPOSITION INFORMATION ON INGREDIENTS

Sodium hypochlorite 5-12.5% and water 87.5-95%
Synonyms: bleach, chlorine bleach

SECTION 3 – HAZARDS IDENTIFICATION

Colorless, slightly cloudy aqueous solution. Bleach odor. Moderately toxic by ingestion and inhalation. Corrosive to body tissues. Avoid contact with body tissues. Strong oxidizing agent.

SECTION 4 – FIRST AID

Call a physician or poison control center.
Inhalation: Remove to fresh air immediately. Give artificial respiration of breathing has stopped.
Eye or external exposure: Immediately flush the area with fresh water at least15 minutes.
Internal/Ingestion: Rinse mouth. Give large quantities of water to dilute. Contact physician or poison control center immediately.

SECTION 5 - FIREFIGHTING

Triclass, dry chemical extinguisher. Fire risk if contacts organic materials. Emits toxic fumes when heated. Wear PPE and respirators.

SECTION 6 - SPILLS AND ACCIDENTAL RELEASE

Ventilate area and restrict access by unprotected people. Contain spill with sand or absorbent material and store in sealed bag or container.

SECTION 7 – HANDLING AND STORAGE

Store with inorganics bromates and chlorates. Keep container tightly sealed.

SECTION 8 – PPE

Avoid contact with eyes, skin, clothes. Wear chemical splash goggles, chemical-resistant gloves and apron.

SECTION 9 – CHEMICAL AND PHYSICAL PROPERTIES

Colorless, slightly cloudy liquid. Bleach odor. Basic pH.

SECTION 10 – STABILITY AND REACTIVITY

Avoid excessive heat, reducing agents, mineral acids

FIGURE 6-1. MSDS for bleach (sodium hypochlorite) describes key properties of bleach, its hazards, and appropriate safety precautions in the following sections:

1. Chemical product identification: name of chemical and manufacturer, **2.** Ingredients: identifies the specific ingredients of the chemical, **3.** Hazard identification: describes the known health hazards of the chemical, **4.** First aid: identifies first aid measures in case of exposure, **5.** Firefighting: Special precautions and information regarding firefighting, **6.** Spills: how to handle chemical spills, **7.** Handling and storage: safe storage, **8.** PPE required for safe handling, **9.** Chemical and physical properties of the chemical, **10.** Stability and reactivity of the chemical.

Source: Pearson Education/PH College.

require prior approval from management. Because highly toxic substances such as carcinogens and reproductive toxins pose elevated risk, the plan will identify those substances in the workplace and describe standard operating procedures for them.

The plan should describe steps to take if an employee is exposed to hazardous chemicals, including the procedures for consulting medical assistance. The plan will also provide a means for recordkeeping related to training and incidents.

The chemical safety plan also must designate a **chemical hygiene officer** or committee that will establish the safety plan as an official part of safe workplace practice.

WORK SAFE!
Know Workplace Chemical Hazards

Chemicals in your work environment are tools, and like other tools they must be handled and stored safely. You may not use these chemicals yourself at all times, but they will be used and stored in your workplace. Chemicals can cause harm by direct contact with skin and mucous membranes or by inhalation of vapors. Others are flammable, highly reactive, or explosive. Your supervisor will ensure that chemical hazards are communicated in the workplace by labeling chemicals, establishing safe work practices and PPE policies, and providing MSDS and training. Ultimately, it is your responsibility to use these resources to protect yourself and coworkers.

Hazardous Chemicals in the Workplace

Certain diagnostic procedures, medical instruments, and medical treatments employ hazardous chemicals. Healthcare workers must know how to prevent exposure to these hazards. This section focuses on chemicals commonly found in various healthcare settings.

Latex

Latex is a natural rubber product that can trigger allergy in some people. Latex exposure usually occurs through contact with **latex gloves** or inhalation of latex powder. The latex can trigger allergic reactions that become more severe with subsequent exposure; latex gloves with powder trigger worse symptoms. Reactions include skin rashes; hives; eye, nose, and throat allergy symptoms; and asthma. Shock is rare, is associated with severe allergy, and can be fatal.

Latex allergies can be avoided by reducing the use of latex gloves or by using alternatives such as **nitrile gloves** when possible. See Table 6-2 ■ for information on the health effects of latex and how to reduce latex exposure.

Mercury

Mercury is a neurotoxin with acute as well as chronic effects, depending on the exposure. Chronic effects may be irreversible. Much atmospheric mercury originates from the incineration of medical waste that contains mercury from dental amalgams, broken thermometers and sphygmomanometers, and other instruments. Because inorganic elemental mercury, the form in these instruments, has no odor, it can remain undetected in the work environment. Moreover, mercury vapor can be inhaled or absorbed through mucous membranes and skin, so exposure requires no direct contact. See Table 6-3 ■ for information on the health effects of mercury and how to reduce exposure.

TABLE 6-2. Exposure to Latex in the Healthcare Setting

Route of Exposure	Protective Work Practice	Personal Protective Equipment	Signs and Symptoms of Exposure
Skin contact with latex, usually gloves, or inhalation of latex powder	If allergic to latex, avoid contact with latex gloves and areas with latex powder (e.g., storerooms), alert employer, wear medical alert bracelet	Use alternatives such as nitrile gloves instead of latex gloves	Skin rash, hives, itching, flushing, nasal, eye, throat, sinus inflammation, asthma, and shock

Source: NIOSH Alert: *Preventing Allergic Responses to Natural Rubber Latex in the Workplace.* Department of Health and Human Services (NIOSH). Publication No. 97-135.

TABLE 6-3. Exposure to Mercury in the Healthcare Setting

Route of Exposure	Protective Work Practice	Personal Protective Equipment	Signs and Symptoms of Exposure
Inhalation or skin contact following broken sphygmomanometer or thermometer	Replace mercury-containing instruments with aneroid when possible; make spill kits available	None required; If exposed, wear gloves for cleanup, wash skin with soap and water, or flush eyes	Short-term: Headache, cough, chest pain, chest tightness, difficulty breathing, soreness of mouth, tooth loss, nausea, diarrhea Long-term: Shaking of hands, eyelids, lips, jaw, tongue; skin rash; headache; sores in mouth; sore gums; insomnia; excessive salivation; personality changes; irritability; memory loss; indecision; intellectual deterioration

Source: 2010. *NIOSH Pocket Guide to Chemical Hazards.* Department of Health and Human Services (NIOSH).

WORDS OF WARNING!
Prevent Exposure to Mercury

The most effective way to prevent exposure to mercury is to completely replace it. Mercury is no longer necessary for most applications. Mercury blood pressure devices (i.e., sphygmomanometers) account for most of the mercury in healthcare workplaces. These and mercury thermometers should be replaced with equally effective mercury-free equipment such as aneroid sphygmomanometers and alcohol-based or digital thermometers. If mercury-based devices remain in use at your workplace, you must familiarize yourself with the location and use of mercury spill clean-up kits.

The chief risk for mercury exposure for healthcare workers is from broken sphygmoma-nometers and thermometers. Spills should be cleaned up immediately using commercially available mercury spill kits. Exposed materials should be placed in sealed containers for safe storage before disposal. Exposed skin must be washed with soap and water immediately; exposed eyes must be immediately flushed with water for at least 15 minutes. The area of the healthcare setting where the spill occurred should be well ventilated to disperse vapor.

Glutaraldehyde

Glutaraldehyde is used to disinfect medical instruments that cannot be heat sterilized. For example, glutaraldehyde is used to disinfect instruments with lenses, including endoscopes; bronchoscopes; ear, nose, and throat instruments; and some other surgical instruments. Glutaraldehyde is also used to fix tissue samples in pathology labs and as a hardening agent in the development of x-rays. Glutaraldehyde causes asthma and skin allergies, and is an eye irritant. It is a colorless, oily, pungent liquid, most often in aqueous solutions of 1 to 50% under trade names Cidex®, Sonacide®, Sporicidin®, Hospex®, Omnicide®, Metricide®, and Wavicide® (Figure 6-2).

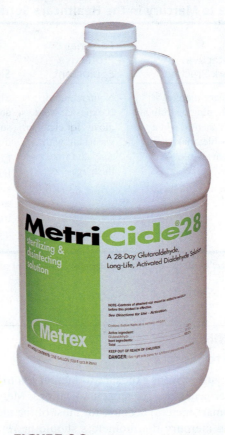

FIGURE 6-2.

Metricide. Brand name of a commonly used formulation of glutaraldehyde.

Source: Metrex, Orange, California.

TABLE 6-4. Exposure to Glutaraldehyde in the Healthcare Setting

Route of Exposure	Protective Work Practice	Personal Protective Equipment	Signs and Symptoms of Exposure
Inhalation and through skin during disinfection of surgical instruments and surfaces, while fixing tissues for pathology, during x-ray development	Use local exhaust ventilation at point of use and keep glutaraldehyde baths used for disinfection under a fume hood if possible, use the minimal volume required for disinfection, wash gloved hands after handling glutaraldehyde, seal or cover all containers holding glutaraldehyde solutions, attend training classes in safety awareness about use of and exposure to glutaraldehyde	Avoid skin contact: Use gloves and aprons made of nitrile or butyl rubber (latex gloves do not provide adequate protection); wear goggles and face shields	Throat and lung irritation, asthma, breathing difficulty, wheezing, nose irritation and sneezing, epistaxis (nosebleed), burning eyes and conjunctivitis, contact and allergic dermatitis, staining hands brown, hives, headache, nausea

Source: Glutaraldehyde: Occupational Hazards in Hospitals. Department of Health and Human Services NIOSH Publication No. 2001-115.

Healthcare workers using glutaraldehyde may protect themselves with good work practices and protective equipment. See Table 6-4 ▪ for information on the health effects of glutaraldehyde and how to reduce exposure.

Ethylene Oxide

Ethylene oxide is a colorless gas used in healthcare settings for sterilizing medical equipment. Ethylene oxide exposure occurs through inhalation, eyes, and skin, causing acute problems such as eye pain and difficulty breathing. Long-term exposure to small amounts is linked to cancer. In fact, the National Institute for Occupational Safety and Health (NIOSH) recommends handling ethylene oxide as a potential carcinogen, and the American Conference of Governmental Industrial Hygienists (ACGIH) classifies it as a carcinogen. An OSHA standard on ethylene oxide applies to a workplace (the **Ethylene Oxide standard**) if the workplace produces amounts above a certain threshold. Most healthcare workplaces do not reach that threshold, so they fall under the Occupational Exposure to Hazardous Chemicals Laboratory standard. Fortunately, it is possible to control exposure to ethylene oxide. See Table 6-5 ▪ for information on the health effects of ethylene oxide and how to reduce exposure.

Bleach

Bleach is a solution of sodium hypochlorite. Applying a 10% aqueous solution for 10 minutes is useful for disinfecting surfaces. However, bleach emits an offensive odor, and the liquid and vapor both irritate skin and mucous membranes. Bleach is not frequently used in the healthcare workplace.

TABLE 6-5. Exposure to Ethylene Oxide in the Healthcare Setting

Route of Exposure	Protective Work Practice	Personal Protective Equipment	Signs and Symptoms of Exposure
Inhalation, skin absorption, eyes	Replace ethylene oxide with other sterilizing practices if possible	Impervious clothing, gloves, aprons, and chemical splash goggles to prevent skin and eye contact	Short-term: Nausea, headache, weakness, vomiting, drowsiness, uncoordination, eye irritation; skin contact causes blisters, burns, edema, frostbite, dermatitis Long-term: Skin sensitization, numbing of sense of smell, respiratory infections; ethylene oxide is a suspected carcinogen

Source: 1998. Occupational Safety and Health Guideline for Ethylene Oxide Potential Human Carcinogen. Department of Health and Human Services (NIOSH).

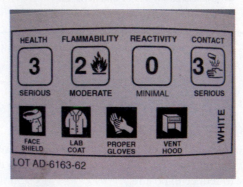

FIGURE 6-3.
Hazard warning on formalin label.

Source: Pearson Education/PH College.

Formaldehyde

Formaldehyde is a colorless gas with an irritating, pungent odor. **Formalin** is the aqueous solution of 10 to 50% formaldehyde containing methanol stabilizer (Figure 6-3). The chief related concern for healthcare workers is exposure to formalin used for preserving tissues and embalming. Exposure occurs through inhalation and skin, causing allergic responses such as asthma and dermatitis or eczema. Exposure to formaldehyde, a carcinogen, has been linked to nasal and lung cancer. Healthcare workplaces using formaldehyde that reaches certain levels fall under the **Formaldehyde standard**. See Table 6-6 ■ for information on the health effects of formaldehyde and how to reduce exposure.

Hazardous Drugs and Anticancer Agents

Healthcare workers may be exposed to a variety of **anticancer agents**, antiviral drugs, chemotherapy agents, hormones, and other **hazardous drugs**. These toxic drugs, depending on exposure, can cause skin rashes, infertility, miscarriage, birth defects, leukemia, or other cancers. Exposure typically occurs through skin following contact with the drugs, or via bodily fluids, urine, and feces containing these drugs. See Table 6-7 ■ for information on reducing exposure to these drugs.

This discussion is not comprehensive. Instead, this chapter focuses on the main hazardous chemicals likely encountered in healthcare workplaces. Healthcare workers must take responsibility and learn about workplace hazards. They should begin by reading the MSDS for each chemical and asking employers for assistance in identifying and preventing exposure to chemical hazards.

TABLE 6-6. Exposure to Formaldehyde in the Healthcare Setting

Route of Exposure	Protective Work Practice	Personal Protective Equipment	Signs and Symptoms of Exposure
Inhalation, skin absorption, eyes	Label formaldehyde bottles "potential cancer hazard," attend training classes in safety awareness about use of and exposure to formaldehyde	Impervious clothing, gloves, aprons, and chemical splash goggles to prevent skin and eye contact with formaldehyde	Eye and throat irritation, coughing, wheezing; subsequent exposures may trigger severe allergic reactions in skin, eyes, respiratory system (asthma)

Source: OSHA Fact Sheet: Formaldehyde. Occupational Safety and Health Administration. www.osha.gov

TABLE 6-7. Exposure to Hazardous Drugs and Anticancer Agents in the Healthcare Setting

Route of Exposure	Protective Work Practice	Personal Protective Equipment	Signs and Symptoms of Exposure
Skin contact with drugs or urine, or feces containing drugs	Wash hands with soap and water immediately before and after using PPE, use syringes and IV sets with Luer-Lok fittings for preparing and administering hazardous drugs, place drug-contaminated syringes and needles in chemotherapy sharps containers for disposal, handle hazardous wastes and contaminated materials separately from other trash, clean and decontaminate work areas before and after each activity involving hazardous drugs and at the end of each shift, clean up small spills of hazardous drugs immediately, using proper safety precautions and PPE	Disposable gown made of polyethylene-coated polypropylene material (which is nonlinting and nonabsorbent); gown should have a closed front, long sleeves, and elastic or knit closed cuffs; do not reuse gowns; face shield when splashes to the eyes, nose, or mouth may occur	Varies, depending on drug, amount, and route of exposure. Consult MSDS and NIOSH List of Hazardous Drugs

Source: NIOSH Alert: *Preventing Occupational Exposures to Antineoplastic and other Hazardous Drugs in Health Care Settings.* Department of Health and Human Services (NIOSH) Publication No. 2004-165.

NIOSH List of Antineoplastic and Other Hazardous Drugs in Healthcare Settings 2010. Department of Health and Human Services (NIOSH).

Chapter Summary

- OSHA Standards protect healthcare workers from exposure to hazardous chemicals.
- Healthcare workers can use safe work practices and PPE to protect themselves and patients from hazardous chemicals commonly found in their workplace.
- A chemical hygiene and safety plan guides the safety policies and procedures at the workplace.
- Employers should train employees to recognize and avoid chemical hazards.

Application

Case Study 6-1: Anticancer Agents in Ambulatory Oncology Clinics

Medical assistants, nurses, and office staff working in ambulatory oncology clinics have increased risk of exposure to hazardous anticancer drugs. They may be exposed directly to these medications or to bodily fluids containing the medications or their metabolites. A routine procedure in oncology clinics is disposal of patient urine samples.

Questions:

1. Describe personal protective equipment for handling this urine.
2. Describe a safe work practice while performing this task.

Case Study 6-2: Latex Allergy

Your coworker is allergic to latex and cannot wear latex gloves. She asked your supervisor to purchase a substitute so that she can safely protect her hands during work. Your supervisor obtained hypoallergenic latex gloves, but these gloves triggered allergic symptoms, too.

Questions:

1. Why did your coworker react to hypoallergenic latex gloves?
2. What sort of gloves can she safely wear?

Assessment

Select the one best answer.

1. Which chemical is used for disinfection in the healthcare setting?
   a. glutaraldehyde
   b. iodine
   c. alcohol
   d. bleach
   e. all of the above

2. _____ is a toxic flammable gas used to sterilize surgical and dental instruments.
   a. ethylene oxide
   b. formaldehyde
   c. alcohol

d. bleach

e. all of the above

3. The best way to prevent exposure to mercury is _____.

   a. wear gloves and mask while using blood pressure devices

   b. ventilate rooms where mercury is used

   c. replace thermometers and blood pressure devices that contain mercury

   d. regularly clean surfaces of examination rooms

   e. all of the above

4. The most effective replacement for latex gloves is _____.

   a. hypoallergenic latex gloves

   b. low powder latex gloves

   c. nitrile gloves

   d. cotton gloves

   e. none of the above

5. Where can you find all of the information about a chemical's properties and hazards?

   a. standard operating procedures for using the chemical

   b. the chemical's MSDS

   c. the chemical hygiene plan

   d. the chemical container's label

   e. none of the above

Resources

Glutaraldehyde: Occupational Hazards in Hospitals. National Institute for Occupational Health and Safety Publication No. 2001-115. Department of Health and Human Services 2001

National Research Council www.nationalacademies.org/nrc

NIOSH Alert: *Preventing Allergic Responses to Natural Rubber Latex in the Workplace.* Publication No. 97-135. Department of Health and Human Services 1997

NIOSH Alert: *Preventing Occupational Exposures to Antineoplastic and Other Hazardous Drugs in Healthcare Settings.* Publication No. 2004-165. Department of Health and Human Services 2004

NIOSH List of Antineoplastic and Other Hazardous Drugs in Healthcare Settings. National Institute for Occupational Health and Safety 2010. Department of Health and Human Services.

Occupational Safety and Health Administration www.osha.gov

1978, September. *Occupational Health Guide for Inorganic Mercury.* Department of Health and Human Services, Department of Labor, OSHA.

1988. *Occupational Safety and Health Guideline for Ethylene Oxide Potential Human Carcinogen.* Department of Health and Human Services (NIOSH).

OSHA Fact Sheet: Formaldehyde. Occupational Safety and Health Administration www.osha.gov

CHAPTER 7

Radiation Safety: Best Practices

This chapter introduces best practices for radiation safety and safe handling of radioactive materials used in the healthcare workplace. Protective equipment and standard operating procedures for controlling exposure are also discussed.

Objectives

After completing this chapter, the student will be able to:

- Describe the main sources of radiation exposure in the healthcare workplace.
- Name the agencies responsible for radiation safety in the healthcare workplace.
- List the regulations and guidelines pertaining to radiation safety in the healthcare workplace.
- Describe safe radiodiagnostic and radiotherapy practices.

Key Terms and Concepts

as low as reasonably achievable (ALARA)
brachytherapy
computed tomography (CT)
diagnostic radiotherapy
distance
dose limitations
dosimeter
duration
fluoroscopy
ionizing radiation
justification
National Council on Radiation Protection and Measurements (NCRP)

Nuclear Regulatory Commission (NRC)
optimization
radiation protection actions
radiation protection principles
radioactivity
radiopharmaceutical therapy
shielding
Standards for Protection against Radiation
teletherapy
therapeutic radiation
x-ray

Diagnostic and Therapeutic Procedures

Healthcare workers are exposed to radiation in their workplace, to background environmental radiation, and to radiation used for their own diagnosis and treatment. Thus healthcare workers may be exposed to more radiation than the general patient population. Radiation damages cells and genes, and may cause abnormal cell function, tumors, and cancers. High radiation doses are associated with leukemia and multiple myeloma as well as breast, bladder, colon, liver, lung, esophageal, ovarian, and stomach cancers. Cancers resulting from occupational radiation exposure look like cancers that arise from other causes. That is because the underlying problem in cancer is mutations, which can be induced by both natural and artificial radiation.

Many other factors contribute significantly to the development of cancer, for example, smoking, diet, obesity, and alcohol use. There is little evidence that the low additional doses of radiation that healthcare workers receive at work increase their risk for cancer; lifestyle factors and genetics have a much greater influence on the development of cancer than their incrementally greater workplace exposure to radiation. However, radiologists are conservative and assume that a healthcare worker who has more exposure, no matter how small, also has an incrementally greater risk. For that reason, healthcare workers are advised to take appropriate precautions to reduce their exposure.

Radioactivity

Radioactivity is the process of unstable isotope decay that releases energy as particles or rays. **Ionizing radiation** produces ions when it interacts with atoms. Natural sources of radiation include cosmic rays, gamma rays from the Earth, and radon. Artificial sources include medical x-rays and therapeutic or diagnostic radioactive materials.

Alpha, beta, and gamma radiation and x-rays are ionizing radiation (Figure 7-1). Alpha radiation cannot penetrate the skin but is harmful when inhaled, swallowed, or absorbed through open wounds. Beta radiation may penetrate skin to its germinal layer, where new skin is produced. Therefore, prolonged contact with beta particles injures the skin, and beta particles can also cause injury if they are swallowed or inhaled. Gamma

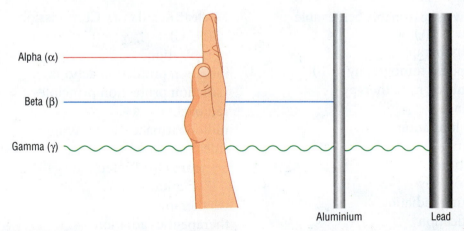

Alpha (α)

Beta (β)

Gamma (γ)

Aluminium   Lead

FIGURE 7-1.
The properties of alpha, beta, and gamma radiation.

TABLE 7-1. Radiation Units of Measurement

Conventional Units	SI Units	Application
roentgen (R)	coulomb/kg	Applies to absorption of gamma rays and x-rays in air.
rad (radiation absorbed dose)	gray (Gy)	The amount of energy deposited per unit weight of human tissue. This is the quantity most directly related to biological effects. Absorbed dose expresses the concentration of radiation energy actually absorbed in tissue.
rem (radiation equivalent man)	sievert (Sv)	The rem is used for specifying biologically equivalent dose and is the traditional measure for biological exposure to radiation after compensating for the type of radiation involved. It is the unit of occupational exposure and biological risk.

radiation travels far through the air and several centimeters in human tissue. Gamma radiation and x-rays pose hazards to surface (skin) as well as to deeper tissues and organs. This is why dense materials such as lead are used to provide a shield from gamma radiation.

Units of Radiation Exposure Two systems measure radiation exposure. The conventional system is the most familiar one in use in the United States. The International Standard (SI) system is based on the metric system and provides a unified system for radiologists (Table 7-1 ■). Even so, the conventional units continue to be used by the radiology community.

Radiation Uses in the Workplace Diagnostic radiotherapy or **therapeutic radiation** is used on nearly one third of all patients admitted to hospitals and is commonly used in outpatient facilities. Diagnostic uses of radiation include **x-rays, computed tomography (CT),** and **fluoroscopy**. Radioactive materials are also ingested, inhaled, or injected, and the photons released are detected using a gamma camera to visualize organ structure and function. For example, radioactive iodine permits imaging the thyroid gland, and other radioisotopes are used to form images of bone, blood circulation, and some organs.

Therapeutic radiation is administered using **teletherapy**, **brachytherapy**, and **radiopharmaceutical therapy.** These procedures expose patients to various doses of radiation with the intent to selectively shrink, damage, or kill diseased tissue, tumors, or cancer. Table 7-2 ■ describes diagnostic and therapeutic procedures that use radiation.

Radiation Regulations

The **Nuclear Regulatory Commission (NRC)** regulates the safe use of radioactive materials in the healthcare workplace. Applicable federal standards are found in the NRC's **Standards for Protection against Radiation.** In addition, the NRC publishes guidelines for radiation in the healthcare workplace in *Regulatory Guide: Information Relevant to Ensuring That Occupational Radiation Exposures at Medical Institutions Will Be as Low as Reasonably Achievable*. In the United States, 38 states are designated Agreement States, which indicates that they have entered into an

TABLE 7-2. Diagnostic and Therapeutic Uses of Radiation

X-ray and CT	X-rays pass through tissues of the body, the amount depending on the radio-density of the various tissues, and form pictures on a computer or television monitor. A radiologist views and interprets the images. An x-ray is performed with a standard x-ray machine or with a computer-aided machine, a CT machine.
Fluoroscopy	Uses x-rays to form real-time images of the structure and function of internal structures and organs. Fluoroscopy may be used in conjunction with surgery.
Radionuclide diagnostics	Radioactive material is injected, inhaled, or ingested. The radiopharmaceutical collects in the organ or area being evaluated, where it emits photons that are detected using a gamma camera. The gamma camera images provide information about the organ function and composition, and help healthcare providers determine organ size, locate and identify tumors, and assess organ function. Technetium-99m is used in the diagnosis of bone, heart, or other organ disorders. Radioactive iodine is used for imaging the thyroid gland.
Teletherapy	An intense beam of radiation from a powerful source is focused on cancerous tissue. An example of teletherapy is the use of a device called the Gamma Knife, which focuses radiation from cobalt-60 sources to a specific location deep within brain tissue.
Brachytherapy	Lower level radioactive sources are placed close to, or within, cancerous tissue, such as in the breast, prostate, or cervix. Sources include sealed small packets called seeds injected or surgically implanted, then removed after the patient receives the prescribed dose. Intravascular brachytherapy systems use small sources that are placed into arteries via catheters.
Radiopharmaceutical therapy	In therapeutic nuclear medicine, high dosages of radioactive materials are injected into, or ingested by, the patient. One example is the use of radioactive iodine to destroy or shrink a diseased thyroid.

Sources: Nuclear Regulatory Commission. 2008. *Fact Sheet: Medical Use of Radioactive Materials.* www.nrc.gov
Health Physics Society. 2010. *Radiation Exposure from Medical Exams and Procedures.* www.hps.org

agreement with the NRC to regulate their radioactive materials. The list of Agreement States and their regulations can be found at the NRC Website (http://nrc-stp.ornl.gov/rulemaking.html).

The **National Council on Radiation Protection and Measurements (NCRP)** publishes additional guidelines and handbooks about limiting exposure to ionizing radiation and radiation protection principles.

Both Standards for Protection against Radiation and the NRC's Regulatory Guide require an institution to develop a radiation safety plan. The institution must designate a radiation safety officer to enforce regulations and policies regarding radiation. The radiation safety plan and the duties of the radiation safety officer are based on certain radiation protection principles and actions.

The first **radiation protection principle** is **justification**; the benefits of radiation exposure should outweigh the known risks. For example, if therapeutic radiation is used for cancer, clinical evidence must show that the risk from therapy is significantly less than the risk of untreated cancer. The second principle is **optimization,** which includes using doses that are **as low as reasonably achievable (ALARA);** doses should be both effective and ALARA for therapy and diagnosis. That is, the known minimal effective radiation dose should be used. The third principle is **dose limitation;** exposures should be monitored to meet legal occupational dose limitations for healthcare workers and others in the workplace. Recommended exposure limits are set by the U.S. National Council on Radiation Protection (NCRP) and worldwide by the International Council on Radiation Protection. Annual dose limits are:

Whole body: 5,000 millirem (mrem)/year

Lens of eye: 15,000 mrem/year

Extremities, skin, and individual tissue: 50,000 mrem/year

Minors: 500 mrem/year

Embryo/fetus: 500 mrem/9 months

General public: 100 mrem/year

Radiation protection actions, derived from these principles, are described in detail by a radiation safety plan. Radiation protection actions fall into three general areas. First, workers must consider the **duration** of radiation dose because the radiation exposure dose is directly proportional to the time of exposure. Second, **shielding**—usually in the form of lead aprons, portable lead shields, or lead and concrete walls—must be employed to shield workers from radiation exposure. Third, **distance** must be maintained between the radiation source and exposed individuals. Radiation dose is inversely proportional to the square of the distance from the source (Figure 7-2). Doubling the distance from a source reduces the amount of radiation exposure by a factor of 4.

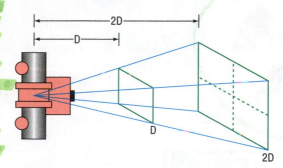

FIGURE 7-2.

Inverse square law. As radiation diverges from an x-ray tube, it covers an increasingly larger area as the distance from the source increases. Doubling the distance from a source reduces the amount of radiation exposure by a factor of 4.

WORK SAFE!
X-Ray Shielding and Viewing Windows

Staff, healthcare providers, or family members may view a patient during x-ray examination if he or she is properly shielded. Each person in the x-ray examination room must wear a lead apron. When watching a patient from an adjacent viewing room, the clear plastic or glass window provides protection because the windows are manufactured with lead mixed into the plastic or glass.

Reducing Radiation Exposure

It is beyond the scope of this book to describe detailed safe operating procedures for x-ray, CT, fluoroscopy, teletherapy, brachytherapy, radiopharmaceutical therapy, and other nuclear medicine procedures. This chapter reviews general radiation safety practices applicable to most radiation procedures and of interest to healthcare workers who would like to know how to reduce occupational radiation exposure.

Equipment design barriers and protective gear are of special importance for radiation protection because radiation cannot be detected by sight, sound, or odor, and safe work

---

WORDS OF WARNING!
Hazard Signs

Heed warnings when you see them in the workplace. Radioactive material must be labeled, and areas where radioactive materials are handled must be identified. The NRC requires the trefoil symbol be posted where radioactivity may be present. In addition, other signs may communicate more about the potential hazards.

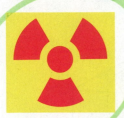

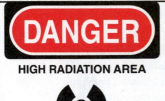

1. Trefoil   2. The caution banner sign

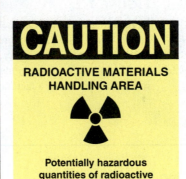

3. The danger sign   4. The caution sign

Source: Environmental Protection Agency

practices alone cannot afford protection. Still, barriers and protective gear coupled with certain work practices can reduce occupational exposure to be consistent with the ALARA principle.

Diagnostic X-Ray, CT, and Fluoroscopy Precautions

These precautions are consistent with the NRC standards and are aimed at maintaining occupational radiation exposure ALARA.

1. Only essential personnel, the radiologist or technician, should be in the x-ray room during patient exposure. Parents and family members may be permitted to join the patient if they stay with healthcare personnel in the protected x-ray machine control booth throughout the exposures. If not in the protected booth during exposure, personnel and family members must wear protective aprons.

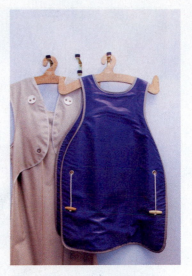

FIGURE 7-3.
Lead apron for chest, abdomen, and pelvis protection.
Source: Gusto/Science Source.

2. Room doors should be closed during exposure to prevent scattered radiation from entering surrounding areas.

3. Personnel should not hold patients during exposure. If the patient must be assisted, the assistant should be nonradiology staff and should wear a protective apron (Figure 7-3) during exposure.

4. All personnel working with radiation sources must wear personal **dosimeters** (Figure 7-4) when working in the radiology department, when using radiographic equipment, and when handling radioactive materials.

5. When performing fluoroscopy, personnel must wear protective aprons and stand several steps away from the patient, 1 to 3 meters if possible.

6. When using mobile x-ray equipment, personnel should stand as far away as possible, as permitted by electric cords (2 meters), from x-ray equipment. Personnel must wear protective aprons or use a protective shield and direct the x-ray beam at the patient only.

Radiopharmaceutical Precautions

Diagnostic radiopharmaceuticals may be injected, ingested, or inhaled. Radiopharmaceuticals may also be administered therapeutically. A comprehensive description of precautions is not possible here. The following describes precautions that apply to the handling of this sort of radioactive material and will be of interest to both radiology and nonradiology personnel. These precautions are also derived from NRC guidelines for reducing occupational exposure.

1. All workers handling radioactive materials should always use shielding materials (syringe shields, gloves, aprons, and lead shields as needed), maintain as much distance as possible from radiation sources, and limit the time of exposure to radiation sources to the time necessary to carry out the required task or clinical procedure.

A
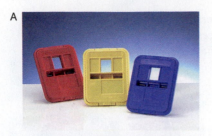

B
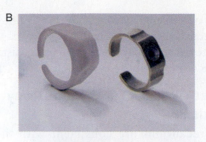

C
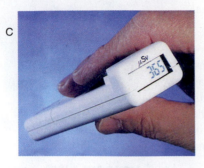

D
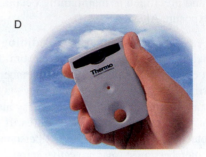

FIGURE 7-4.

Radiation dosimeters. (A) Film badge. (B) Finger ring. (C) Pocket dosimeter.
(D) Whole body dosimeter.

Source: (A–C) PTW-New York Corporation, (D) Health Protection Agency/Science Source.

2. Radioactive sources should be handled only with tongs or tweezers and protective gloves (Figure 7-5).
3. Workers who handle containers of radioactive materials must wear finger dosimeters and body dosimeters, except when handling low-level radioactive sources that produce a dose rate of less than 5 mrem/hr at 1 cm distance.
4. Nursing staff and others working with patients who may be excreting radioactive material must follow precautions to avoid contaminating themselves and others.
5. Exposed personnel must avoid contaminating the patient environment, light switches, sink taps, or doorknobs.
6. Radioactive solutions should never be pipetted by mouth.
7. Eating, smoking, drinking, and applying cosmetics should be prohibited in laboratories where radioactive materials are handled.
8. Special precautions should be taken to avoid the possibility of small amounts of radioactive material entering cuts.
9. The use of containers or glassware with sharp edges should be avoided. Care should be taken to avoid bites or scratches in working with animals to which radioactive materials have been administered.
10. Food and drink should not be stored in the same place (e.g., refrigerator) with radioactive materials.
11. Radioactive materials should be placed in a locked room when personnel are not present.

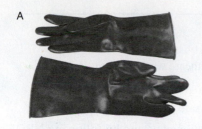
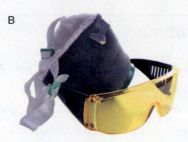

FIGURE 7-5.

Shielding equipment. (A) Protective gloves. (B) Eyewear.

Source: (A) Lloyd Fudge/Fotolia (B) Fotolia.

Chapter Summary

- Diagnostic and therapeutic procedures expose healthcare workers to radiation.
- NRC regulations guide safe radiation practices.
- Radiation protection principles and actions inform safe practices.
- Healthcare workers can reduce occupational radiation exposure by following NRC guidelines.

Application

Case Study 7-1: X-Ray Safety

At the pediatric clinic where you work, parents are occasionally asked to help hold their child still during an x-ray exam. When parents help, you give them a lead apron to wear. Sometimes they question the need to wear an apron.

Questions:

1. Do the parents need to wear a lead apron? Explain why.
2. Parents are exposed to a small amount of radiation. What is the concern?

Case Study 7-2: Brachytherapy Concerns

Some patients at the cancer treatment clinic where you work receive brachytherapy. One patient is concerned about sharing the waiting room with other patients who are "radioactive" because they have been receiving brachytherapy.

Questions:

1. Are patients who are receiving brachytherapy "radioactive"?
2. What precautions should patients and staff take?

Assessment

Select the one best answer.

1. As you move farther from a radiation source, the amount of radiation you are exposed to _____ .
   a. increases
   b. decreases
   c. remains the same
   d. cannot be determined

2. The radiation protection principles include _____ .
   a. dose limitation
   b. optimization and ALARA
   c. justification
   d. all of the above
   e. none of the above

3. Which form of radiation travels far in air and penetrates several centimeters into tissues?
   a. alpha
   b. beta
   c. gamma
   d. all of the above
   e. none of the above

4. Radioactive iodine taken orally to treat thyroid cancer is an example of _____ .
   a. fluoroscopy
   b. teletherapy
   c. radiopharmaceutical therapy
   d. brachytherapy

5. When applying ALARA, healthcare workers should always _____ .
   a. minimize the amount of exposure time
   b. use shielding
   c. use the lowest effective radiation dose
   d. work at greatest practical distance from the radiation source
   e. all of the above

Resources

Health Physics Society. 2010. *Radiation Exposure from Medical Exams and Procedures.* www.hps.org

National Council on Radiation Protection and Measurements. *Limitation of Exposure to Ionizing Radiation (Supersedes NCRP Report No. 91),* Report No. 116. www.ncrp.org

Nuclear Regulatory Commission. *10 CFR Part 20 Standards for Protection against Radiation.* www.nrc.gov

Nuclear Regulatory Commission. 2008. *Fact Sheet: Medical Use of Radioactive Materials.* www.nrc.gov

Nuclear Regulatory Commission. *Regulatory Guide 8.18: Information Relevant to Ensuring That Occupational Radiation Exposures at Medical Institutions Will Be as Low as Reasonably Achievable.* www.nrc.gov

GLOSSARY

13 Carcinogens Standard: OSHA standard applicable to manufacturing, processing, repackaging, release, handling, or storage of 13 carcinogens

administrative controls: work procedures and safe work practices set by the employer, including written safety policies and rules, designated supervision, recordkeeping, and training programs

AIDS: acquired immunodeficiency syndrome, caused by the human immunodeficiency virus (HIV)

airborne infection isolation room: specially ventilated room with negative air pressure

airborne precautions: infection control measures that prevent transmission of pathogens known to be transmitted through the air in small droplets

ALARA: *see* as low as reasonably achievable; radiation safety principle that advocates keeping exposure to radiation as low as reasonably achievable

alcohol: chemical disinfectant often used in hand soaps, lotions, or hand-rubs

American National Standards Institute: nongovernmental agency that provides guidelines for the manufacture of safety equipment

ANSI: *see* American National Standard Institute

antiretroviral medication: drugs used to control HIV infections

antibiotic resistance: the ability of certain bacteria to survive the effects of antibiotics that normally would kill them

antibodies: protective proteins secreted by lymphocytes in response to infections

anticancer agents: a class of therapeutic and potentially toxic chemicals used to treat cancer

antigens: substances derived from pathogens that trigger an immune response

as low as reasonably achievable: radiation safety principle, ALARA, advocates for minimizing radiation exposure as much as possible

bacteria: single-celled prokaryotic organisms

blood-borne pathogens: infectious agents transmitted in blood and body fluids; usually refers to HIV, hepatitis B virus, and hepatitis C virus

Bloodborne Pathogens Standard: OSHA standard applicable to workplaces with occupational exposure to blood-borne pathogens such as HIV, hepatitis B, and hepatitis C

brachytherapy: therapeutic placement of low-level radioactive sources within cancerous tissue

catheter-associated urinary tract infections: infectious diseases transmitted during catheterization of the urethra, often abbreviated as CAUTIs

CAUTIs: *see* catheter-associated urinary tract infections

chain of infection: describes the route and means of transmission of a pathogen from an infected host to another susceptible host

chemical hazard: chemicals that pose threats to human health

chemical hygiene officer: an employee charged with implementing and enforcing a chemical hygiene and safety plan

chemical hygiene plan: document describing safe work practices, as well as safe storage, handling, and disposal of hazardous chemicals

chlorhexidine gluconate: disinfectant for hand hygiene or surgical scrub

cirrhosis: liver damage and scarring triggered by hepatitis or alcoholism

Clinical Laboratory Improvement Amendments: provide oversight and regulation for safe and accurate performance of certain clinical laboratory tests

CLIA: Clinical Laboratory Improvement Amendments prescribe training for certain laboratory tests and procedures to ensure safety and reliability of tests

CLIA-waived: Laboratory tests that do not require special CLIA-approved training

communicable diseases: infectious diseases transmitted directly from one person to another

computed tomography: computer-assisted x-ray imaging technique

contact precautions: measures taken to reduce exposure to pathogens transmitted primarily by direct contact

CT: computed tomography, a type of x-ray imaging

Department of Energy: federal agency that provides standards for working with radioactive materials

Department of Labor: federal agency in which OSHA resides

diagnostic: a procedure used for the purpose of identifying the nature of a disease

diagnostic radiotherapy: the use of radioactive materials to determine the nature of a disease

dialysis: treatment for kidney disease that involves drawing blood from a vein, removing toxins and metabolic waste, and returning the blood directly into a vein

distance: a principle of radiation exposure; as distance increases, exposure decreases

distance principle: a radiation protection principle based on increasing the distance from a radioactive source to reduce exposure

dose limitation: a principle of radiation safety that advocates using the smallest therapeutic dose possible

dosimeter: a device that measures exposure to radioactivity

droplet precautions: measures taken to reduce exposure to pathogens transmitted mainly in respiratory droplets

duration: a principle of radiation exposure; as duration increases, exposure increases

duration principle: a radiation protection principle based on decreasing the time of exposure to a radioactive source

engineering controls: the safety practice of creating facilities, equipment, and work processes that eliminate hazards from the work environment

ethanol: *see* alcohol

ethylene oxide: toxic gas used for sterilizing medical equipment

Ethylene Oxide standard: OSHA standard applicable to workplaces with occupational exposure to ethylene oxide

exposure control plan: describes procedures and controls for limiting exposure to blood-borne pathogens

fluoroscopy: imaging method that uses x-rays to form real-time images of the structure and function of internal structures and organs

fomite: an inanimate object capable of transmitting infectious diseases

formaldehyde: colorless toxic gas mixed with methanol to preserve and harden tissue specimens

Formaldehyde standard: OSHA standard applicable to workplaces with occupational exposure to formaldehyde

formalin: aqueous solution of 37 to 50% formaldehyde-containing methanol stabilizer

fungi: eukaryotic organisms, including yeast, molds, mushrooms

glutaraldehyde: colorless, oily pungent liquid disinfectant used on medical instruments, tissue fixative, x-ray developing fluid

HAI: *see* healthcare-associated infection

hand hygiene: infection control measures that include hand washing and use of gloves; includes hand rubbing with alcohol-based antiseptics

hazard communication: use of signs, reports, labels, and training to prevent exposure to hazards in the work environment

Hazard Communication standard: OSHA standard describing safe practices for handling, labeling, and disposing of hazardous chemicals

hazardous chemicals: Chemical substances that are flammable, caustic, explosive, or may cause biological damage

hazardous drugs: medications that cause cell damage or death or may be radioactive

HBV: *see* hepatitis B virus

HCV: *see* hepatitis C virus

healthcare-associated infections: infectious diseases transmitted to patients by healthcare personnel, procedures, or equipment

helminths: flatworms and roundworms

hepatitis B vaccine: highly effective and safe vaccine that protects an individual from hepatitis B infections

hepatitis B virus: blood-borne virus that causes acute and sometimes chronic liver infection

hepatitis C virus: blood-borne virus that causes chronic and serious liver infection

HIV: *see* human immunodeficiency virus

human immunodeficiency virus: the retrovirus that causes AIDS

immune compromised: a condition of weakened immunity

infectious disease: communicable disease caused by pathogenic microorganisms

intravascular catheter–associated bloodstream infections: infectious diseases of the blood transmitted during catheterization of veins

iodine: chemical disinfectant often used on skin

iodophor: iodine-containing disinfectant often used on skin

ionizing radiation: radiation such as x-rays with enough energy to damage DNA and proteins

Ionizing Radiation standard: radiation such as x-rays and gamma rays with enough energy to cause atoms to lose electrons (to ionize)

isopropanol: *see* isopropyl alcohol

isopropyl alcohol: rubbing alcohol used to disinfect skin surfaces

justification: a radiation protection principle that states the benefits of therapeutic radioactive substances should outweigh potential harm of not using these substances

latex: natural rubber product used in manufacture of gloves

latex gloves: protective, disposable gloves made from the rubber compound latex

lymphocytes: white blood cells that help to protect the body from infection

material safety data sheet (MSDS): describes a chemical's properties and hazards

mercury: a neurotoxic element used in thermometers and sphygmomanometers

methicillin-resistant *Staphylococcus aureus*: a strain of *Staphylococcus aureus* that cannot be treated with the antibiotic methicillin

mode of transmission: describes how an infectious disease is passed from one person to another

MRSA: *see* methicillin-resistant *Staphylococcus aureus*

National Council on Radiation Protection and Measurements (NCRP): an agency that define safe use, storage, and disposal of radioactive susbstancces

nitrile gloves: protective, disposable gloves made from nitrile butadiene rubber, a nonlatex alternative for people with latex allergy

nosocomial infections: also known as healthcare-associated infections, these infections are transmitted to patients by healthcare personnel, procedures, or equipment

notifiable diseases: infectious diseases that must be reported to the Centers for Disease Control and Prevention (CDC)

n-propanol: alcohol used as a topical antiseptic or disinfectant

Nuclear Regulatory Commission (NRC): a government agency of the U.S. Department of Energy, the NRC regulates the use of radioactive materials

Occupational Exposure to Hazardous Chemicals in the Laboratory Standard: OSHA standard applicable to all workplaces with occupational exposure to hazardous chemicals

Occupational Radiation Protection standard: Department of Energy standard applicable to the safe use of radioactive materials in the workplace

Occupational Safety and Health Administration: an agency in the U.S. Department of Labor, OSHA prescribes and enforces standards for workplace safety

opportunists: microorganisms that cause disease in weakened or immune-compromised hosts or in damaged tissues and organs

optimization: a radiation protection principle that states therapeutic and diagnostic radiation should be used at doses that maximize therapy while minimizing side effects and risks for hazards

OSHA: *see* Occupational Safety and Health Administration

pathogen: a disease-causing microorganism

pathogenic: the ability of a microorganism to cause disease

PPE *see* personal protective equipment

personal protective equipment (PPE): safety equipment such as eyewear, respirators, goggles, gloves and aprons or gowns worn to provide a barrier to hazards when other safety controls are inadequate

polaxamer: a topical antiseptic

portal of entry: the site at which a pathogen enters the body

portal of exit: the site at which a pathogen leaves the body

postexposure prophylaxis: treatment following possible or known exposure to an infectious disease

povidone: iodine-containing disinfectant often used on skin surfaces

protozoa: microscopic, single-celled eukaryotic organisms

radiation hazard: risk to human health caused by exposure to radioactive materials

radiation protection actions: safety practices that minimize exposure to harmful radiation; these include minimizing doses and use of protective barriers

radiation protection principles: safety principles that guide safe practice; these ALARA—keeping doses as low as reasonable achievable

radioactivity: the process of unstable isotope decay that releases energy as particles or rays

radionuclide diagnostics: use of radioactive chemicals for diagnostic and imaging purposes

radiopharmaceutical therapy: use of radioactive chemicals for therapeutic purposes

reservoir: the natural source of a pathogen

resident flora: microorganisms normally living in or on the human body

respiratory and cough etiquette: infection control measures aimed at controlling pathogens transmitted by coughing and sneezing

safe injection practice: procedure for safe use and disposal of needles and catheters

safe work practice: established safe work procedures developed to protect workers from hazards

shielding: using a barrier that blocks radioactivity

SSI: *see* surgical site infection

standards: minimal safety guidelines

standard operating procedure: work procedure established for all employees to protect workers from hazards

standard precautions: infection control measures that include hand hygiene, contact precautions, airborne precautions, droplet precautions, and safe injection practices

Standards for Protection against Radiation: Nuclear Regulatory Commission standards applicable to the safe use of radioactive materials in the healthcare workplace

surgical site infection (SSI): infection acquired in surgical skin wounds

susceptible host: a person who is capable of being infected

teletherapy: therapeutic radiation procedure in which an intense beam of radiation from a powerful source is focused on cancerous tissue

therapeutic radiation: use of radiation for treatment

tissue: a collection of cells that share similar structure and function as well as embryonic origin

tissue graft: a tissue or organ surgically introduced to the body

transient flora: microorganisms that transiently reside in or on the body

transmission-based precautions: infection control measures that block the specific and known routes of transmission for an infectious disease

universal precautions: infection control measures used at all times in all settings to prevent infection by blood-borne pathogens

urinary tract infection (UTI): usually healthcare-associated infection of the urethra, ureter, or kidney

UTI: *see* urinary tract infection

vaccination: a procedure in which a substance is injected to stimulate immunity to a specific pathogen

vancomycin-resistant enterococci (VRE): colon or vaginal bacteria that have evolved resistance to the antibiotic vancomycin

VAP: *see* ventilator-associated pneumonia

vector: an animal, often an insect, that transmits infections

ventilator-associated pneumonia (VAP): hospital-acquired infection associated with use of ventilators

virus: intracellular pathogen

VRE: *see* vancomycin-resistant enterococci

worms: small, simple animals that infest intestines or blood

x-ray: diagnostic imaging technique that utilizes the radioactive energy of x-rays

APPENDIX A

Nationally Notifiable Infectious Conditions

The following infections must be reported to the Centers for Disease Control and Prevention (CDC), which tracks the incidence of these diseases.

Anthrax

Arboviral neuroinvasive and non-neuroinvasive diseases
- California serogroup virus disease
- Eastern equine encephalitis virus disease
- Powassan virus disease
- St. Louis encephalitis virus disease
- West Nile virus disease
- Western equine encephalitis virus disease

Botulism
- Botulism, foodborne
- Botulism, infant
- Botulism, other (wound and unspecified)

Brucellosis

Chancroid
Chlamydia trachomatis
Cholera
Cryptosporidiosis
Cyclosporiasis

Dengue
- Dengue fever
- Dengue hemorrhagic fever
- Dengue shock syndrome

Diphtheria

Ehrlichiosis/Anaplasmosis
- *Ehrlichia chaffeensis*
- *Ehrlichia ewingii*
- *Anaplasma phagocytophilum*
- Undetermined

Giardiasis

Gonorrhea
Haemophilus influenzae, invasive disease
Hansen disease (leprosy)

Hantavirus pulmonary syndrome
Hemolytic uremic syndrome, postdiarrheal

Hepatitis

- Hepatitis A, acute
- Hepatitis B, acute
- Hepatitis B, chronic
- Hepatitis B perinatal infection
- Hepatitis C, acute
- Hepatitis C, chronic

HIV

- HIV infection, adult/adolescent (age greater than or equal to 13 years)
- HIV infection, child (age greater than or equal to 18 months and less than 13 years)
- HIV infection, pediatric (age less than 18 months)

Influenza infection in children that results in mortality

Legionellosis
Listeriosis
Lyme disease
Malaria
Measles
Meningococcal disease
Mumps
Novel influenza A virus infections
Pertussis
Plague
Poliomyelitis, paralytic
Poliovirus infection, nonparalytic
Psittacosis

Q Fever

- Acute
- Chronic

Rabies

- Animal
- Human

Rubella

Rubella, congenital syndrome
Salmonellosis
Severe acute respiratory syndrome–associated Coronavirus (SARS-CoV) disease

Shiga toxin-producing *Escherichia coli* (STEC)
Shigellosis
Smallpox
Spotted fever rickettsiosis
Streptococcal toxic-shock syndrome
Streptococcus pneumoniae, invasive disease

Syphilis

- Primary
- Secondary
- Latent
- Early latent
- Late latent
- Latent, unknown duration
- Neurosyphilis
- Late, non-neurological
- Stillbirth
- Congenital

Tetanus

Toxic-shock syndrome (other than Streptococcal)
Trichinellosis (Trichinosis)
Tuberculosis
Tularemia
Typhoid fever
Vancomycin, intermediate *Staphylococcus aureus* (VISA)
Vancomycin, resistant *Staphylococcus aureus* (VRSA)
Varicella (morbidity)
Varicella (deaths only)
Vibriosis

Viral hemorrhagic fevers

- Arenavirus
- Crimean-Congo hemorrhagic fever virus
- Ebola virus
- Lassa virus
- Marburg virus

Yellow fever

Source: Centers for Disease Control and Prevention (CDC). *Nationally Notifiable Infectious Conditions,*
United States 2010. www.cdc.gov

APPENDIX B

Healthcare-Associated Infections

Infection	
Acinetobacter baumannii	Cause: bacteria
	Signs and symptoms: respiratory infection resembles bacterial pneumonia; wound infection occasionally develops necrotizing fasciitis
	Patient treatment: antibiotics (carbapenems, polymyxins, tigecycline)
	Hospital transmission: direct contact; respiratory infection associated with tracheostomy or ventilator, infects open wounds
	Infection control measures: hand hygiene, environmental hygiene
	Special notes: resistant to multiple antibiotics; uncommon infection, occurs mostly among immune-compromised and older adults; the pathogen earned the name *Iraqibacter* because of increased incidence among wounded soldiers in Iraq
Burkholderia cepacia	Cause: bacteria
	Signs and symptoms: respiratory infection resembles pneumonia
	Patient treatment: co-trimoxazole (trimethoprim/sulfamethoxazole)
	Hospital transmission: direct contact; respiratory infection occurs with chronic lung disease and cystic fibrosis
	Infection control measures: hand hygiene
	Special notes: transmission has been documented via contaminated nasal sprays, mouth washes, sublingual thermometers; antibiotic resistant; the bacteria have been cultured from betadine and chlorhexidine mouthwash

Infection	
Chickenpox (Varicella)	Cause: varicella virus
	Signs and symptoms: red spotted rash that blisters and dries; low fever; weakness; mild respiratory symptoms
	Patient treatment: symptomatic
	Hospital or ambulatory care transmission: direct contact, respiratory droplets, and aerosolized virus from skin lesions
	Infection control measures: hand hygiene, use gloves during patient contact; vaccination for healthcare personnel who have no serologic proof of immunity, no prior vaccination, or history of varicella disease
Clostridium difficile (also called C- diff)	Cause: bacteria
	Signs and symptoms: watery diarrhea and abdominal pain, nausea; may develop pseudomembranous colitis, a severe colon infection
	Patient treatment: if antibiotic-associated, then antibiotic treatment must be stopped; severe cases require metronidazole or vancomycin
	Hospital transmission: endospores and bacteria shed in feces, transmitted by contaminated hands and surfaces
	Infection control measures: hand hygiene with soap and water (alcohol ineffective against the endospores), use gloves during patient contact, hypochlorite-based disinfection of surfaces, disinfection of endoscopes, isolation of patients, judicious use of antibiotics
	Special notes: risks include antibiotic exposure (especially long-term use of fluoroquinolones), gastrointestinal (GI) surgery, long stay in healthcare setting, serious underlying illness, immune-compromised condition, advanced age

Clostridium sordellii	Cause: bacteria Signs and symptoms: gynecologic and postpartum infection with hypotension and leukocytosis Patient treatment: beta-lactams, clindamycin, tetracycline and chloramphenicol Hospital or ambulatory transmission: unknown; *C. sordellii* colonizes vagina in 29% of women after abortion; *C. sordellii* is detected in vaginal secretions of 5 to 10% of non-pregnant women Infection control measures: unknown; presumably hand hygiene and surface/environmental hygiene Special notes: most infections occur in women following live births or abortions; postpartum infections have extremely high mortality
Gastrointestinal (GI) infections	Cause: various bacteria and viruses Signs and symptoms: depends on cause but may include fever, abdominal pain, diarrhea, vomiting Patient treatment: usually only supportive treatment and rehydration because often the diseases are self-limiting Hospital, ambulatory, and home care transmission: contact with feces and contaminated materials, food, water Infection control measures: hand hygiene Special notes: relatively rare in hospitals
Hepatitis A	Cause: hepatitis A virus Signs and symptoms: jaundice, nausea, vomiting, fever, abdominal pain, weakness Patient treatment: usually self-limiting Hospital, ambulatory, and home care transmission: contact with feces and contaminated materials Infection control measures: avoid eating and drinking in patient areas; hand hygiene; vaccine not routinely recommended unless healthcare worker has regular occupational exposure Special notes: uncommonly acquired in hospitals; usually acquired from patients with undiagnosed hepatitis or with severe diarrhea

Infection	
Hepatitis B	Cause: hepatitis B virus
	Signs and symptoms: jaundice, nausea, vomiting, fever, abdominal pain, weakness; may become chronic infection and may lead to cirrhosis or liver cancer
	Patient treatment: antiviral medications, including adefovir dipivoxil, interferon alfa-2b, pegylated interferon alfa-2a, lamivudine, entecavir, telbivudine
	Hospital and ambulatory care transmission: contaminated needles, needle-stick injuries, contact with wounds and blood
	Infection control measures: vaccination, standard precautions
	Special notes: most adults recover completely and do not become chronically infected; up to 50% of children between the ages of 1 and 5 years become chronically infected; the incidence of hepatitis B has dropped dramatically (annual occupational infections decreased 95%) since the introduction of the vaccine in 1982
Hepatitis C	Cause: hepatitis C virus
	Signs and symptoms: jaundice, nausea, vomiting, fever, abdominal pain, weakness
	Patient treatment: pegylated interferon and ribavirin; HCV is leading indication for liver transplants in the United States
	Hospital and ambulatory care transmission: contaminated needles, needle-stick injuries, contact with wounds and blood; transfusions and transplants rarely cause HCV
	Infection control measures: standard precautions; no vaccine available
	Special notes: 75 to 85% will develop chronic infection, 60 to 70% will develop chronic liver disease, 5 to 20% will develop cirrhosis over a period of 20 to 30 years, and 1 to 5% will die from liver cancer or cirrhosis

HIV/AIDS	Cause: human immunodeficiency virus
	Signs and symptoms: early infection may include flu-like illness; recurrent opportunistic infections, including pneumocystis pneumonia, tuberculosis, candidiasis, diarrhea, Kaposi's sarcoma, weight loss
	Patient treatment: antiretroviral therapy (ART) is a combination therapy that includes two nucleosides (e.g., AZT and ddI) plus a protease inhibitor (e.g., indinavir) or two nucleosides plus a non-nucleoside reverse-transcriptase inhibitor (e.g., efavirenz); patients also receive preventive care and treatment for opportunistic infections and AIDS symptoms
	Hospital and ambulatory care transmission: contaminated needles, blood and body fluid contact with open skin wound, eyes, mouth, nose; the risk for occupationally acquired HIV is extremely low
	Infection control measures: use standard precautions; postexposure prophylaxis depends on severity of exposure (e.g., cutaneous versus deep needle-stick injury) and on HIV status of source (positive or unknown) and may require ART with two or three drugs); no vaccine available
Influenza	Cause: influenza virus
	Signs and symptoms: fever, headache, sore throat, muscle aches, fatigue, cough; may become complicated by bacterial or viral pneumonia, bronchitis, ear and sinus infections
	Patient treatment: no specific treatment usually required because infection is usually self-limiting; persons at high risk or with severe symptoms may require antiviral drugs such as oseltamivir (Tamiflu®) and zanamivir (Relenza®)
	Hospital, ambulatory, and home care transmission: large respiratory droplets from coughing and sneezing
	Infection control measures: hand hygiene, cough etiquette, vaccination
	Special notes: healthcare workers usually acquire seasonal flu in the community

Infection	
Intravascular catheter–associated bloodstream infections	Cause: variety of skin bacteria Signs and symptoms: fever, cardiovascular shock Patient treatment: antibiotics Hospital transmission: skin bacteria introduced to blood via intravenous catheter Infection control measures: hand hygiene, gloves, catheter site preparation and hygiene Special notes: fairly uncommon but associated with high morbidity, longer hospital stays, and increased medical costs
MRSA: Methicillin-resistant *Staphylococcus aureus*	Cause: bacteria Signs and symptoms: in the healthcare setting, MRSA causes bloodstream infections, surgical site infections, and pneumonia, with signs and symptoms that vary with site of infection; in the community, most MRSA infections are skin infections associated with skin trauma and abrasions Patient treatment: skin infections require incision, drainage, and antibiotic treatment guided by the organism's susceptibility profile Hospital and ambulatory care transmission: contact with skin, wounds, contaminated body fluids Infection control measures: standard precautions, contact precautions, environmental hygiene, patient isolation, screening high-risk patients Special notes: high-risk patients include those with weakened immune systems; high-risk procedures include surgery and catheterizations

Norovirus	Cause: norovirus
	Signs and symptoms: diarrhea, vomiting, stomach pain
	Patient treatment: no specific treatment; rehydration therapy
	Hospital transmission: fecal-oral route
	Infection control measures: hand hygiene; during patient contact use gloves; environmental hygiene; use contact precautions with incontinent patients; environmental disinfection requires bleach; quaternary ammonium compounds on utensils may not be effective; heat disinfection to 140° F is effective; no vaccine
	Special notes: highly contagious, requiring as few as 100 norovirus particles for infection
Pneumonia	Cause: various bacteria and viruses
	Signs and symptoms: chest pain, cough, fever, weakness, symptoms vary with the cause; chest x-ray and sputum cultures are diagnostic
	Patient treatment: antibiotics for bacterial pneumonia; no specific treatment for viral pneumonia
	Hospital transmission: ventilators, intubation, contact with contaminated hands, mainly ventilator-associated
	Infection control measures: hand hygiene, respiratory and intubation equipment sterility, disinfection
	Special notes: accounts for 15% of hospital-acquired infections, the second most common; 27% of all intensive care unit (ICU) infections; 20 to 33% mortality
Surgical site infection	Cause: skin, respiratory, or GI bacteria
	Signs and symptoms: depending on site, pus, redness, swelling, necrosis, fever
	Patient treatment: may require incision, drainage, and antibiotics
	Hospital transmission: contact with skin or respiratory bacteria such as staphylococci or with GI bacteria
	Infection control measures: standard pre- and postsurgical precautions that include disinfection, surgical scrub, and personal protective equipment (PPE), including gowns, masks, gloves; postoperative wound hygiene
	Special notes: Relatively rare

Infection	
Tuberculosis (TB)	Cause: bacteria, *Mycobacterium tuberculosis*
	Signs and symptoms: cough, bloody sputum, fever, chills, night sweats, chest pain, weight loss, fatigue
	Patient treatment: latent infections are treated with isoniazid for 9 months; active infections are treated with isoniazid, rifampin, ethambutol, or pyrazinamide for 6 to 12 months
	Hospital transmission: mainly respiratory droplets from infected patients; also during bronchoscopy and sputum collection
	Infection control measures: TB screening of staff and of patients at risk; isolation of infected patients, hand hygiene, masks, gloves, disinfection of bronchoscopes; prompt treatment of diagnosed patients
	Special notes: usually transmitted by patients with undiagnosed TB
Urinary tract infections	Cause: various skin or colon bacteria
	Signs and symptoms: pain during urination, cloudy or bloody urine, fever
	Patient treatment: antibiotics
	Hospital transmission: nearly all transmitted during catheterization
	Infection control measures: evaluate catheter use and reduce use when possible; hand hygiene, gloves; skin disinfection before procedure
	Special notes: 30% of all hospital-acquired infections, the most common

VISA: Vancomycin-intermediate *Staphylococcus aureus* and VRSA: Vancomycin-resistant *Staphylococcus aureus*	Cause: bacteria, *Staphylococcus aureus*
	Signs and symptoms: in the healthcare setting, VISA and VRSA cause bloodstream infections, surgical site infections, and pneumonia, with signs and symptoms that vary with site of infection
	Patient treatment: VISA and VRSA are treatable with a variety of antibiotics
	Hospital, ambulatory, and home care transmission: contact with skin, wounds, contaminated body fluids
	Infection control measures: standard precautions, contact precautions, environmental hygiene, patient isolation, screening high-risk patients
	Special notes: high-risk patients include those with weakened immune systems; high-risk procedures include surgery and catheterizations
VRE: Vancomycin-resistant enterococci	Cause: bacteria, *Enterococcus faecalis* or *E. faecium*
	Signs and symptoms: varies by site of infection and may include urinary tract infections, wound infections, or catheter-associated wound infections
	Patient treatment: most infections can be treated with antibiotics other than vancomycin
	Hospital, ambulatory, or home care transmission: contact with skin, surgical wounds, catheterization
	Infection control measures: hand hygiene, standard precautions, contact precautions, judicious antibiotic use
	Special notes: occurs mostly among immune-compromised patients and after abdominal or chest surgery

Source: Centers for Disease Control and Prevention www.cdc.gov

APPENDIX C

Reproductive Health and Safety

Reproductive problems such as infertility, miscarriage, and low birth weight are prevalent in the general population and are not exclusively linked to the healthcare workplace. For example, 1 in 6 pregnancies end in miscarriage, 2 to 3% result in major birth defects, 7% in low birth weights, 10% in developmental delays and disorders, and 10 to 15% of couples remain infertile after one year of trying to bear children. This high background prevalence makes it difficult to link reproductive problems to the workplace. Yet these data suggest that healthcare workers should consider reducing any known additional reproductive health risks associated with work.

The effects of reproductive hazards vary and depend on the nature and timing of exposure. Reproductive hazards during the first 3 months of pregnancy might cause a birth defect or a miscarriage. During the last 6 months of pregnancy, exposure to reproductive hazards could impair growth of the fetus, affect organ development, or induce premature delivery. Thus it is important to know these hazards and avoid them early in family planning and throughout pregnancy.

Infectious Hazards Pregnant women and fetuses are at no greater risk for acquiring pathogens, but the potential for infections to seriously affect reproductive health requires vigilance and precaution. Several viruses, including blood-borne pathogens, should be avoided because of their effects during pregnancy. In general, the infection control practices described in Chapter 4 also apply to pregnant healthcare workers.

Infectious Reproductive Hazards

Pathogen	Effects on Reproductive Health	Exposure	Prevention
Cytomegalovirus	Birth defects, low birth weight, developmental disorders	Healthcare workers in contact with infants and children	Hand hygiene
Hepatitis B virus	Low birth weight	All healthcare workers exposed to blood and body fluids	Vaccination and standard precautions
Human immunodeficiency virus (HIV)	Low birth weight, childhood cancer	All healthcare workers exposed to blood and body fluids	Standard precautions
Human parvovirus B19	Miscarriage	Healthcare workers in contact with infants and children	Hand hygiene
Rubellavirus (German measles)	Birth defects, low birth weight	Healthcare workers in contact with infants and children	Vaccination before pregnancy if no prior immunity

(continued)

(continued)

Pathogen	Effects on Reproductive Health	Exposure	Prevention
Varicella-zoster virus (chickenpox)	Birth defects, low birth weight	Healthcare workers in contact with infants and children	Vaccination before pregnancy if no prior immunity

Sources: 1999. National Institute for Occupational Safety and Health. *The Effects of Workplace Hazards on Female Reproductive Health*. Publication No. 99-104, Department of Health and Human Services. 1996. National Institute for Occupational Safety and Health. *The Effects of Workplace Hazards on Male Reproductive Health*. Publication No. 96-132, Department of Health and Human Services.

Chemical and Physical Hazards Chemical and physical hazards in the healthcare setting mainly include anticancer agents, mercury, and radiation. All chemicals must be treated with respect because the reproductive hazards of all chemicals remain unknown. Good chemical hygiene practices (Chapter 6) apply to pregnant workers. These practices include the following:

1. Use personal protective equipment (gloves, respirators, and personal protective clothing) to reduce exposures to workplace hazards.
2. Ensure that chemicals are stored in sealed containers when they are not in use.
3. Perform hand hygiene after contact with hazardous substances and before eating, drinking, or smoking.
4. Avoid skin contact with chemicals.
5. If chemicals contact the skin, follow the directions for washing in the material safety data sheet (MSDS).
6. Review all MSDS to become familiar with any reproductive hazards used in your workplace. If you are concerned about reproductive hazards in the workplace, consult your healthcare provider.
7. Participate in all safety and health education, training, and monitoring programs offered by your employer.
8. Learn about proper work practices and engineering controls (such as improved ventilation).
9. Prevent home contamination:
   - Change out of contaminated clothing and wash with soap and water before going home.
   - Store street clothes in a separate area of the workplace to prevent contamination.
   - Wash work clothing separately from other laundry (at work if possible).
   - Avoid bringing contaminated clothing or other objects home; if work clothes must be brought home, transport them in a sealed plastic bag.

Physical and Chemical Reproductive Hazards

Hazard	Effects on Reproductive Health	Exposed Workers
Anticancer agents	Infertility, miscarriage, birth defects, low birth weight	Healthcare workers caring for cancer patients
Mercury vapor	Abnormal sperm, impaired male sexual performance, birth defects, developmental disorders	Healthcare workers exposed to broken mercury instruments
Ionizing radiation (e.g., x-rays)	Infertility, miscarriage, birth defects, low birth weight, developmental disorders, childhood cancers	Healthcare workers and dental personnel

*Sources:*1999. National Institute for Occupational Safety and Health. *The Effects of Workplace Hazards on Female Reproductive Health.* Publication No. 99-104, Department of Health and Human Services.
1996. National Institute for Occupational Safety and Health. *The Effects of Workplace Hazards on Male Reproductive Health.* Publication No. 96-132, Department of Health and Human Services.

Resources for Reproductive Health and Safety

1999. National Institute for Occupational Safety and Health. *The Effects of Workplace Hazards on Female Reproductive Health.* Publication No. 99-104, Department of Health and Human Services.

1996. National Institute for Occupational Safety and Health. *The Effects of Workplace Hazards on Male Reproductive Health.* Publication No. 96-132, Department of Health and Human Services.

Pregnancy and Universal Precautions. Centers for Disease Control and Prevention (CDC). www.cdc.gov

Radiation Exposure and Pregnancy. June 2010. Health Physics Society. www.hps.org

INDEX

Note: Page references followed by "f," "t," and "b" denote figures, tables, and boxes, respectively.